Promoting a Fighting Spirit

Linda Seligman

· ·

Promoting a Fighting Spirit

Psychotherapy for
Cancer Patients, Survivors,
and Their Families

Jossey-Bass Publishers
San Francisco

Substantial discounts on bulk quantities of Jossey-Bass books are available to corporations, professional associations, and other organizations. For details and discount information, contact the special sales department at Jossey-Bass Inc., Publishers. (415) 433–1740; Fax (800) 605–2665.

For sales outside the United States, please contact your local Simon & Schuster International office.

 Manufactured in the United States of America on Lyons Falls Pathfinder Tradebook. This paper is acid-free and 100 percent totally chlorine-free.

Library of Congress Cataloging-in-Publication Data

Seligman, Linda.
    Promoting a fighting spirit : psychotherapy for cancer patients, survivors, and their families / Linda Seligman.
        p.   cm.
    Includes bibliographical references and index.
    ISBN 0-7879-0190-3
    1. Cancer—Psychological aspects.   2. Psychotherapy.   I. Title.
RC271.P79S45   1996
616.99'4'0019—dc20   95-32119

FIRST EDITION
HB Printing 10 9 8 7 6 5 4 3 2 1

Contents

• •

Preface

· ·

I am a cancer survivor, the daughter of a father who had colon cancer, the niece of an aunt who had breast cancer, and the niece of two uncles who died of cancer. Cancer has played an important role in my life and that of my family just as it does in the lives of so many people.

As it often is, cancer was not only a source of great shock, pain, and loss in my life but also a source of new perspectives and opportunities. I became increasingly interested in learning how to help people who had been diagnosed with cancer to cope with cancer and its treatments, and I discovered a new and growing body of literature that is encouraging and empowering. Not only can people learn to cope successfully with the emotional impact of cancer but they can make changes that are likely to enhance their immune systems and enable them to live richer, more rewarding lives. My psychotherapy practice, over the years, has increasingly focused on working with cancer survivors and their families. My work with these people has been more enriching than any I have done before; together, we have struggled with the shock of diagnosis, coped with the rigors of treatment, grieved at losses and treatments that failed, and rejoiced at successes.

Because of the prevalence of cancer, nearly all psychotherapists will find themselves working with cancer survivors and their families, whether or not they specialize in counseling people with cancer. The purpose of this book is to integrate the literature on psychotherapy for cancer survivors and to help therapists both understand the important connection between emotions and cancer and acquire the knowledge and skill they need to provide effective psychotherapy to cancer survivors and their families. The book can also be useful to cancer survivors and their families who want to understand what they are going through and help themselves as much as possible.

This book consists of twelve chapters and a Resources section. Chapter One lays the groundwork for the rest of the book by reviewing the research on the relationship between emotions and cancer. Studies of animals and of people have demonstrated that personality, mood, ways of handling stress, and emotional responses to cancer can make a difference in adjustment to the disease as well as in its prognosis. This chapter also presents evidence supporting the belief that changes in lifestyle and attitude can have an impact on both emotional well-being and physical health.

Chapter Two focuses on helping therapists understand the person with cancer. The chapter reviews many of the variables such as age, ethnicity, gender, psychological resources, and family context that are important determinants of people's reactions to cancer.

Standardized assessment of cancer survivors is the subject of Chapter Three. Relevant sections of the *Diagnostic and Statistical Manual of Mental Disorders* are reviewed as are inventories and other tools that can help therapists understand their clients more clearly.

Chapter Four provides an overview of the research on effective psychotherapy for cancer survivors. The chapter discusses the stages in the process of coping with cancer and suggests goals and interventions that psychotherapists might consider for each of those stages.

Cognitive psychotherapy, probably the most important approach to psychotherapy with cancer survivors, is the topic of Chapter Five. This chapter reviews the literature that supports using this approach with cancer survivors and presents information on important cognitive models and techniques including Moorey and Greer's model, the approaches of Aaron Beck and David Burns, Martin Seligman's "learned optimism," visualization, meditation, decision making and problem solving, hypnosis, affirmations, discussion of dreams, and reading and writing.

Chapter Six continues the discussion of approaches to psychotherapy with cancer survivors by focusing on behavioral and affective approaches. Specific behavioral interventions reviewed in this chapter include stress management, relaxation, systematic desensitization, distraction, skill development, biofeedback, activities, and exercise. This chapter also covers the use of expressive therapies, existential psychotherapy, psychodynamic psychotherapy, empathy, and medication.

Chapter Seven provides information on what interventions are effective in helping people deal with particular facets of the diagnosis and treatment of cancer. Interventions are suggested that can ameliorate the negative impact of the diagnosis, surgery and hospitalization, chemotherapy, radiotherapy, other aversive procedures, physical and sexual changes associated with cancer, and cancer-related pain.

The beneficial use of groups for cancer survivors and their families is the topic of Chapter Eight, which provides information on both psychotherapy groups and peer support groups.

Chapter Nine focuses on the impact of cancer on family and interpersonal dynamics. This chapter views cancer survivors in context and discusses ways in which others can be helpful, the impact of cancer on family members as well as on friendships, and the importance of understanding family dynamics and functioning in helping people cope with cancer.

Chapter Ten looks at cancer survivors' relationships with health care providers and psychotherapists and provides guidelines for improving those interactions. This chapter looks at the role of therapists working with these clients and the benefits and challenges of this work. The chapter also discusses the special role of the therapist who is a cancer survivor.

Chapter Eleven focuses on death and recurrence. It reviews fears and feelings associated with a negative outcome to cancer treatment and provides ways to help people with cancer, as well as their friends and family, cope with recurrence, death, and loss.

Chapter Twelve presents information on life as a cancer survivor. Whether people remain cancer-free for a brief period of time or many years, once cancer has been diagnosed, it will almost inevitably have a profound impact. This chapter looks at ways to help people deal with the fear of recurrence, to improve their physical and emotional health, and to make the most of their lives.

The Resources section at the end of this book includes additional tools and information to help cancer survivors and their therapists. It provides an outline of a model for providing short-term psychotherapy to people with a diagnosis of cancer, worksheets that can be used in group or individual psychotherapy, a list of recommended readings for both therapists and their clients, and a list of support groups and other sources of help and information.

Bethesda, Maryland   Linda Seligman
October 1995

Acknowledgments

This book is dedicated to cancer survivors everywhere who are living the material in this book. I especially want to thank the many cancer survivors I have counseled over the years who have contributed their experiences, thoughts, and feelings to this book. I am particularly appreciative of all I learned from T.C., B.G., L.W., M.O., J.M., J.S., C.P., P.C., D.L., J.C., M.J., B.P., L.S., I.S., G.L., P.O., Z.D., R.H., R.D., A.F., R.D., B.S., I.G., G.R., K.M., M.G., J.W., L.C., B.T., and the members of Bosom Buddies.

I would also like to thank Dr. Frederick P. Smith, Dr. Roger J. Friedman, Dr. Garry D. Ruben, and Dr. Robert H. Weinfeld, without whose help this book would not have happened.

Essential to the completion of this book was the help I received from Bonnie Moore and Merle Wexler, doctoral students in counseling in the Graduate School of Education at George Mason University. Their help in gathering sources of information and conducting interviews for this book contributed immeasurably to its quality.

I would like to thank George Mason University for granting me the research leave that enabled me to write this book.

Finally, as always, I would like to thank my husband, Dr. Robert Zeskind, for his support, advice, encouragement, and patience.

L. S.

The Author

LINDA SELIGMAN received her Ph.D. degree in counseling psychology from Columbia University. She is a professor at George Mason University in Fairfax, Virginia, where she is in charge of the graduate program in community agency counseling.

Seligman is a licensed psychologist and licensed professional counselor. She has experience in a variety of clinical settings including psychiatric hospitals, university counseling centers, community mental health centers, substance abuse treatment programs, foster care, corrections, and private practice. She is currently the director of the Center for Counseling and Consultation, a private practice with offices in Fairfax, Virginia, and Bethesda, Maryland.

Seligman's research interests include diagnosis and treatment planning, counseling people with cancer, and career counseling. She is the author of four books, *Assessment in Developmental Career Counseling* (1980), *Diagnosis and Treatment Planning in Counseling* (1986), *Selecting Effective Treatments* (1990), and *Developmental Career Counseling and Assessment* (1994). She has written over forty professional articles and book chapters. In addition, she has lectured throughout the United States and Canada on diagnosis and treatment planning and is a nationally recognized expert on that subject.

Seligman was editor of the *Journal of Mental Health Counseling* and has served as president of the Virginia Association of Mental

Health Counselors. In 1986, she received the Distinguished Faculty Award from George Mason University. In 1990, she was selected Researcher of the Year by the American Mental Health Counselors Association.

Promoting a Fighting Spirit

Emotions and Cancer

T hirty percent of the population of the United States, approximately 75 million people, will have cancer at some time in their lives (Zimpfer, 1992). Three out of four families will need to cope with the impact of cancer. For nearly all of these people, coping with cancer, a chronic as well as a life-threatening illness, will be one of the most frightening and difficult experiences of their lives.

Cancer and its treatment can have a profound impact on emotional adjustment. Approximately half of all people diagnosed with cancer as well as many of their partners will meet the criteria for a mental disorder. Derogatis et al. (1983) found that 47 percent of hospitalized and ambulatory cancer patients they studied had a psychiatric disorder. As many as 25 percent experienced marked psychological dysfunction (Glanz & Lerman, 1992).

The Importance of Counseling People with Cancer

A growing body of literature, most of which has been produced since the middle 1980s, has demonstrated that providing psychotherapy to cancer survivors and their families can have a powerful impact not only on coping and adjustment but also on prognosis.*

---

*The term *cancer survivor* will be used throughout this book because, as Mullan and Hoffman (1990, p. 1) put it, "Survival, quite simply, begins when you are told you have cancer . . . and continues for the rest of your life."

Counseling people with cancer and their families can achieve the following goals:

- Reduce depression and anxiety associated with the diagnosis of cancer while improving coping skills, sense of mastery, and optimism

- Dispel misconceptions and myths about cancer while promoting accurate understanding of the disease and its treatment

- Promote effective communication between cancer survivors and medical staff and help people make sound decisions about treatment

- Reduce pain, nausea, and other aversive consequences of cancer and its treatment

- Encourage development and mobilization of support systems

- Promote positive, helpful communication and cohesiveness within the family unit and reduce stress, confusion, and fear in family members

- Help people to maintain self-esteem despite both short-term and long-term physical changes due to cancer and its treatment

- Establish attitudes and behaviors that may contribute to a more favorable prognosis

- Enable cancer survivors and their families to live a life that is as active and fulfilling as possible for as long as possible

- If necessary, help people cope with recurrence, death, and bereavement

The purpose of this book is to provide therapists from all mental health fields with the information and tools they will need to accomplish these goals with cancer survivors and their families.

The Impact of Stress on the Immune System

Perhaps the most controversial area in the field of psychooncology, the use of psychological principles and techniques to help people cope with cancer, is the area of psychoneuroimmunology. PNI, as it has been called, addresses the direct impact of emotions on disease. In the case of cancer, research has focused primarily on two areas: (1) the relationship of personality and emotions to the incidence and severity of cancer, and (2) the impact that psychosocial interventions have on the course of the disease once cancer has been diagnosed. Although it may seem far-fetched to believe that there is a connection between emotions and cancer, compelling studies of both people and animals are accumulating that provide logical and persuasive evidence of such a connection (Graves, 1990).

Some of the evidence comes from general research on the relationship between stress and illness. The well-known Schedule of Recent Life Events developed by Holmes and Rahe (Kobasa, 1979), for example, assigned points ranging from 1 to 100 to stressful life events (for example, divorce = 73, vacation = 13). People who accumulated total scores of 300 or higher on that scale were much more likely to suffer an illness than people with low total scores.

According to Zimpfer (1992, p. 203), "The mind-body connections seem to proceed on a cause-effect path that is increasingly being recognized as connecting the psychological, neurological, endocrine, and immune systems." A logical explanation of the physiology of this connection can be given. The brain and the immune system are connected through hormones, chemical messengers that can transmit emotional states through the bloodstream from one part of the body to another. When a person experiences stress, the brain signals the brainstem, which in turn excites the visceral autonomic nervous system that regulates body activities. To ready the body for action in response to the stressor, the sympathetic system signals the adrenal glands on each kidney to secrete epinephrine and norepinephrine that will promote rapid movement, the parasympathetic system slows digestion and other functions to ready the body for action, and the pituitary gland at the base of the brain releases endorphins that will further promote an effective response to stress. This readies the body to respond in a fight-or-flight mode but also results in less energy being channeled into the immune system.

While this mobilization of resources is essential to survival, if the stressor is severe and prolonged, particularly if the demands of the stressor exceed the person's coping abilities, the immune system can become depleted. The killer T cells and natural killer (NK) cells that patrol the body through the bloodstream and destroy abnormal cells can lose their effectiveness (Locke & Colligan, 1987). Cancer cells are formed throughout life but normally are detected and destroyed by the immune system. However, when the immune system is impaired, the cancerous cells may gain a foothold and multiply. As Cooper and Watson (1991, p. x) concluded, "Overall, this picture yields more apparent effects showing stress to be associated with cancer than not. The same rationale applies, in somewhat altered form, to progress of cancer."

These findings should not be interpreted to mean that stress or emotional upset is a sufficient or even necessary ingredient of tumor growth. However, in the presence of other factors including carcinogens, a genetic predisposition to cancer, and the sort of personality style that has been associated with cancer, stress can make an important difference in the incidence and prognosis of cancer.

Research Based on Animal Studies

A number of studies have demonstrated a connection between control over stressors and cancer. Visintainer and her colleagues were the first to demonstrate that a psychological state could cause cancer (Visintainer, Volpicelli, & Seligman, 1982). They injected three groups of rats with live tumor cells. Two of the groups were subjected to electric shocks. One group was able to escape from the shocks; the other was not. Among the helpless rats, 73 percent developed cancer. Only 37 percent of the rats who could escape from the electric shocks developed cancer, an incidence not significantly different from that of the control group of rats that did not receive electric shocks. Based on these findings, the authors concluded that stress alone is not the determinant of physiological changes; rather, it is the inability to cope effectively and exert meaningful control over stressful situations.

In a review of subsequent and similar studies, Newberry, Gordon, and Meehan (1991) concluded, "The notion that stressful conditions can alter the development of cancer has been confirmed repeatedly by experiments on animal models" (p. 27) and "Acute, uncontrollable stress is likely to stimulate tumor development, whereas otherwise similar, but controllable, stress is much less likely to have such an effect . . . " (p. 28). In addition, adaption to a stressor or successful experiences in coping with stressors prior to tumor development have been shown in animals to have the potential to prevent stress from having a negative physiological effect.

Research Based on Studies with People

Although thus far the research on the impact of emotions on cancer in people is less clear and conclusive than the animal studies, theoretical and empirical research suggests that three types of risk factors are implicated in the development of cancer in people: (1) stressful experiences, especially early childhood losses; (2) personality styles, especially those characterized by hopelessness, helplessness, passivity, and depression; and (3) personal habits such as smoking or maintenance of a high-fat diet (Redd & Jacobson, 1988).

Probably the most important findings in this area have been those of Greer and his colleagues; Fawzy and Fawzy and their colleagues; Temoshok; Kobasa; and Spiegel and his colleagues.

Personality Style and Health

Kobasa (1979) was one of the first researchers to demonstrate a relationship between personality style and health. Using the Schedule of Recent Life Events developed by Holmes and Rahe, she assessed the extent to which a group of executives had experienced stressful life events over the previous three years. Among those who had experienced high stress, about half had become ill and half had not. In studying the differences between the two groups, Kobasa found that the healthy group demonstrated more of what she called *hardiness*, characterized by "a stronger commitment to self, an attitude of vigorousness toward the environment, a sense of meaningfulness, and an internal locus of control" (p. 1). The three salient characteristics of hardy people are these:

1. A belief that they can exert control over the events in their lives and the confidence that their strengths and resources will enable them to achieve that control

2. An ability to feel deeply involved in or committed to the activities of their lives, a sense of purpose, an involvement with life and other people

3. Ability to view change as an exciting challenge, prizing a life filled with interesting experiences, and the flexibility and resilience that will allow them to cope with the challenges

Kobasa summarized these as control, commitment, and challenge. Although she acknowledged the presence of multiple determinants of the stress-illness connection, including environment, physiological predisposition, early childhood experiences, and socioeconomic resources, Kobasa concluded that personality style was a very important mediator of that connection and could affect a person's chance of becoming ill by as much as 50 percent.

The Relationship of Depression to Cancer

Kobasa's findings have been borne out by other studies. Shekelle, Raynor, and Ostfeld (1981), for example, administered a battery of physiological and psychological tests to a group of over two thousand middle-aged men employed by the Western Electric Company. At follow-up seventeen years later, the only significant predictor of death due to cancer was the Depression Scale of the Minnesota Multiphasic Personality Inventory. In addition, the study found that the higher the level of initial depression, the higher was the risk of death from cancer. This pattern may be explained by the finding that the adrenal glands of depressed people produce large amounts of corticosteroids, which can cause a malfunction in the immune system (Locke & Colligan, 1987).

Temoshok and the Cancer-Prone Personality

The so-called Type A coronary-prone behavior pattern, characterized by such qualities as competitiveness, anger, tension, anxiety, and self-centeredness, has been well established (Temoshok & Dreher, 1992). Temoshok and her colleagues proposed the existence of another behavior pattern, Type C, that was associated with both the risk of developing cancer and recovery from that disease. A humorous yet accurate view of this personality style is reflected by Woody Allen in the film *Manhattan* when he says, "I don't get angry, okay? I mean, I have a tendency to internalize. That's one of the problems I have. I grow a tumor instead" (p. 24).

According to Temoshok and her colleagues (Kneier & Temoshok, 1984; Temoshok & Dreher, 1992), the Type C behavior style is the polar opposite of the Type A pattern and identifies people who tend to be other-directed, have little awareness of their own needs, feel powerless and hopeless, repress anger and other negative emotions, and are reluctant to ask for help. Such people experience little pleasure or enthusiasm and typically are passive, self-sacrificing, and appeasing in their relationships. They often seem depressed and lonely. People with a Type C profile typically come from dysfunctional families where they felt little closeness with their parents and were encouraged to suppress emotion. A history of abuse is frequently reported.

Temoshok and her colleagues also identified a third behavioral pattern they called Type B. People with this behavioral style are able to appropriately express anger as well as other emotions, generally are relaxed and comfortable with themselves, and are capable of both meeting their own needs and responding to others.

Temoshok and Dreher found that among people who had been diagnosed with melanoma, a cancer of the skin, those who were emotionally expressive, the Type A and Type B people, had thinner tumors, more slowly dividing cancer cells, and more signs of immune system effectiveness. Although Temoshok and Dreher, like Kobasa, recognized that cancer was affected by many factors, they concluded that psychological coping might affect the prognosis of the disease by as much as 10 percent. People who are depressed and who have depleted resources, characteristic of a Type C personality, typically react to a diagnosis of cancer with passivity and hopelessness; this process can increase their risk of succumbing to cancer. Temoshok and Dreher further believed that the role of the mind is particularly important in people under age fifty-five when the immune system generally is strong and in certain types of cancer including melanoma, breast cancer, and colon cancer.

Encouraging information provided by Temoshok and her colleagues is the finding that just as Type C behavior can be learned, it can be unlearned. They have developed a model designed to transform a person's Type C behavior so that the person is better characterized by Type B behavior. (This will be discussed further in the section on psychotherapy for people with cancer.) Therapists should bear in mind, then, that behaviors and attitudes that have been associated with a poorer prognosis are amenable to modification. They should also remember that the types described here are prototypes; most people will not be pure types but will have features of several types. People should not be stereotyped but rather should be assessed as individuals. Despite these cautions, the research linking cancer with characteristics of the Type C personality is compelling.

Emotional Response to Cancer and Its Relationship to Prognosis

Greer and Watson (1982) studied the relationship of emotional response to cancer from a different perspective but came up with findings that are very consistent with those of Temoshok and her colleagues. Greer and Watson explored the question of whether the emotional adjustment of people with a diagnosis of cancer could influence the course of the disease. Using the Mental Adjustment to Cancer Scale, they identified four characteristic responses to the diagnosis:

1.   Fighting spirit: People with this reaction fully accepted their diagnosis but were optimistic, sought out information and resources, and were determined to fight the disease.

2.   Positive avoidance (denial): People in this group rejected the diagnosis they received or minimized its seriousness.

3.   Fatalism (stoic acceptance): These people accepted their diagnosis but did not actively seek out information, believing they had no power to influence the course of their disease; they viewed their futures as being in the hands of the medical team or God.

4.   Helpless/hopeless: A belief that their life is over characterized this group of people who felt overwhelmed and consumed by cancer.

A fifth group, characterized by anxious preoccupation with thoughts of the disease as well as feelings of depression, was added as the study progressed.

At five- and ten-year follow-ups, people characterized by a fighting spirit were significantly more likely to be alive and disease-free than those people whose responses had been characterized by fatalism, hopelessness, or extreme emotional distress. Interestingly, the group characterized by denial also had a relatively positive outcome; although people in that group did not have the sense of control and empowerment of the fighting spirit group, their denial of the implications of their disease meant that neither were they consumed by worry and discouragement like the other three groups. This finding seems important for therapists to keep in mind. Denial is not always a negative stance in terms of dealing with cancer; therapists should assess whether the denial is so severe as to seriously impair the person's decision making or whether in fact the denial is helping the person to cope effectively with a very difficult situation.

Both Greer and his colleagues and Temoshok and her colleagues based their research primarily on people who already had received a diagnosis of cancer. Eysenck (1991a) conducted three prospective studies of the link between cancer and personality. He identified the following six personality types:

1. Overcooperative, appeasing, unassertive, reluctant to express negative emotions (Temoshok's Type C)
2. Angry, hostile, aggressive, competitive (Type A)
3. Hysterical, emotionally volatile, and strongly expressive
4. Healthy, autonomous, high in self-esteem
5. Rational, unemotional
6. Egocentric, psychopathic, focused on own needs

Eysenck found that people characterized by the personality configurations in groups 1, 2, and 5 were disease-prone while those in groups 3, 4, and 6 were not disease-prone. In addition, connections between type of disease and personality pattern were found. In a ten-year follow-up, people in group 1 had a significantly higher death rate from cancer than did groups 2, 3, and 4 while those in group 2 had a significantly higher death rate from coronary heart disease than did those in groups 1, 3, and 4. In one persuasive study conducted in Yugoslavia, 50 percent of those in group 1 died of cancer and nearly 30 percent of those in group 2 died of coronary heart disease, while fewer than 5 percent of those in group 4 died of either disease. Eysenck also noted a particularly strong connection between the incidence of cancer and the "number of traumatic life events evoking chronic hopelessness" (p. 78).

Eysenck, like other researchers in this area, recognized the multiplicity of factors inherent in cancer. Nevertheless, he concluded, "Psychosocial variables, and particularly personality type and stress, are important in mediating deaths from cancer and coronary heart disease. These personality variables are more influential than physical factors like smoking, blood pressure, and cholesterol" (p. 82).

A study by Eysenck (1991b) of risk factors for lung cancer shed further light on the cancer-personality connection. Eysenck identified four risk factors for lung cancer: smoking (more than twenty cigarettes a day for at least ten years), heredity (at least one first-degree relative diagnosed with lung cancer), chronic bronchitis, and personality patterns characterized by stress-related responses of helplessness, hopelessness, and depression. The findings indicated that the death rate from lung cancer increased with the number of risk factors, ranging from 0 percent for those with one factor to 31 percent for those with all four factors. Eysenck concluded that risk factors were synergistic and "it is when risk factors combine that they become deadly" (p. 85).

However, Eysenck (1991b), like Temoshok, offered hope. A subsample of those people identified as having the above four factors received behavior therapy. The death rate of those in this subsample was approximately a third as high as in a group of people who had all four factors but who did not receive any psychotherapy.

The Impact of Psychotherapy on People with Early-Stage Cancer

Several other studies have supported the beliefs of Temoshok and Eysenck that psychotherapy can have a beneficial impact on the course of cancer. Fawzy et al. (1993a) randomly divided sixty-eight people with stage I or II (early-stage) malignant melanoma who did not have a major depressive disorder into a control group and an experimental group. Those in the experimental condition were divided into groups of seven to ten participants and received six weekly sessions of ninety-minute group psychotherapy an average of 112 days after surgery. The psychotherapy was designed to be structured and supportive and included information, stress management, enhancement of coping skills, and psychological support.

At six-month follow-up, people in the experimental condition demonstrated significant changes in both physiological and psychological areas. They had reductions in emotional distress and improved use of coping mechanisms. Physiological changes, including an increase in NK cell activity, suggested a strengthening of the immune system. Five to six years after the study began, the control group demonstrated a greater trend toward recurrence and a significantly greater rate of death than the experimental group. Many variables were investigated in this study; however, the only two significant covariables were the depth of the malignant lesion and the group intervention.

Fawzy et al. also found that "higher levels of baseline distress as well as baseline coping and enhancement of active-behavioral coping over time were predictive of lower rates of recurrence and death" (1993, p. 681). The association between higher levels of coping and better medical outcomes had been anticipated. However, the association between higher *initial* distress and better medical outcomes was a surprising and important finding.

Several possible explanations have been offered for these relationships. Those people with higher initial and enhanced coping mechanisms may have done better medically because of the responsiveness of NK cells to psychological intervention and a greater sense of personal control and optimism. However, initially high coping skills, particularly when combined with group psychotherapy, also could have fostered better health habits (for example, improved nutrition, use of sun protection), treatment compliance, and better physician-patient relationships along with better attitudes, stress reduction, a greater sense of social support, and better coping skills. The association between *low* levels of initial distress and a *poorer* prognosis may reflect minimization or avoidance of the seriousness of the condition and consequently poorer health and coping behaviors.

This study has several important implications for therapists and cancer survivors:

1.   Further support is given to the association between prognosis and coping skills, whether initial level or level enhanced by psychotherapy is considered.

2.   However, research has not yet demonstrated conclusively how much if any of the association between strong coping skills and positive prognosis is due to direct physiological effects; some or all of the association may be due to enhanced health care. In fact, 25 percent of the studies on the relationship between emotion and cancer have been inconclusive (Watson & Ramirez, 1991).

3.   Therefore, although the role of psychotherapy in helping cancer survivors both physically and emotionally is well established, psychotherapy should be recommended *in addition to* medical treatment. To suggest that therapy substitute for conventional medical treatment is clearly not indicated and is potentially very dangerous.

4.   Finally, therapists can reassure their clients that initial high distress in response to a diagnosis of cancer is not only understandable and common but also may be a positive prognostic indicator. Having a fighting spirit and strong coping skills may not prevent people from being frightened and upset by a diagnosis of cancer.

However, good coping skills can protect people from being immobilized by their fears. If anything, distress may impel people with a fighting spirit to make even more successful use of the coping skills they already have.

The Impact of Psychotherapy on People with Metastasized Cancer

Most of the research on the relationship between coping style and cancer has focused on cancer survivors with a relatively good prognosis. However, David Spiegel (1992) presented some findings that suggest a connection also exists between psychological variables and the course of advanced cancer. Other than his work, most of the information available on that connection comes from anecdotal writing such as that of Lawrence LeShan (1989) and Bernie Siegel (1990, 1993). Although their descriptions of what Siegel called "exceptional cancer patients" is compelling, they have a magical, too-good-to-be-true quality about them.

David Spiegel, initially skeptical of the idea that psychological factors could bear any relation to cancer prognosis, developed a carefully designed study intended to gather more conclusive and empirical data on that connection. Spiegel (1992) randomly assigned eighty-six women with metastatic (advanced) breast cancer to one of two groups. The women in the experimental group participated in weekly supportive/expressive group therapy for up to a year in addition to their medical treatment. The therapy groups were designed to help the women improve their quality of life, face and deal with their fears, communicate effectively with their physicians, clarify their values and priorities, and control their pain. The women in the control group received only routine medical care.

In a short-term follow-up, the women in the therapy condition reported less tension, fatigue, confusion, and depression and more energy and better coping responses than those who had not had the group experience. After ten years, Spiegel found that the women in

the control group had lived an average of 18.9 months after joining
the study while those in the experimental group had lived an average of 36.6 months after joining the study. Three of the women in
the experimental group were still alive while all those in the control group had died.

Other research supports Spiegel's findings. Grossarth-Maticek
and Eysenck (1989) also studied women with metastatic breast cancer and came up with similar findings. Their study focused on
women in four treatment conditions: those who received no treatment survived an average of 11.28 months, those who received
chemotherapy alone survived an average of 14.08 months, those
who received psychotherapy alone survived an average of 14.92
months, and those who received both chemotherapy and psychotherapy apparently benefited from the synergistic combination
of those two interventions and survived an average of 22.40
months. Psychotherapy not only enhanced survival time but was
also associated with improvement in signs of immune system functioning.

Spiegel's explanations of his findings were similar to those of
other researchers. He acknowledged the possibility of a direct benefit to the immune system of the enhanced coping skills of the
women in the experimental condition. However, he stated with
more assurance that changes in attitudes among those women may
have led to greater compliance with medical recommendations and
improved health behaviors while pain reduction may have allowed
those women to be more active and in that way to achieve a healthier lifestyle.

A new finding emphasized by Spiegel is the importance of social
support. He concluded that social support, especially support that
increased a person's sense of control and assertiveness, seemed to
buffer stress, enabled people with cancer to manage their lives better, and improved medical outcome.

Although these findings are very encouraging, Spiegel raised a
concern about their interpretation. "An internal sense of control

over cancer can be viewed as a two-edged sword. On one hand, people generally associate mastery and positive coping with an inner sense of control. On the other hand, when one is confronted with a progressive and possibly fatal illness, a sense of inner control can be damaging by inducing self-blame for events over which one has no control" (1992, p. 116). Therapists should be careful that cancer survivors do not develop the belief that if only they develop the right psychological attitudes and behaviors, they can cure themselves of cancer. Such a belief is likely to engender guilt and anxiety as well as subvert compliance with recommended medical treatment. Psychological factors, while demonstrably important in determining prognosis, are only some of many factors that influence the course of the disease. A fine balance is important; cancer survivors should be encouraged to take responsibility for themselves, to gather information, and to use effective coping and decision-making skills but should not be made to feel that they alone have control over their disease.

Relationship Between Lifestyle and Cancer

In addition to those studies that examined the correlation between personality and cancer, a group of studies is available that looks at the relationship between lifestyle and health. Berkman and Syme (1979), for example, conducted a nine-year study of seven thousand residents of Alameda County, California. They found that those who were single or widowed, had few friends or family, and participated little in community activities were much more likely to die of cancer than those with extensive personal ties. Only the one factor, termed *isolation-depression*, significantly predicted which people would die of cancer within the nine years following the data collection (Berkman & Breslow, 1983). This was true regardless of income, gender, race, ethnicity, and age.

Ell, Nishimoto, Mediansky, Mantell, and Hamovitch (1992), too, found a connection between lifestyle and cancer. They found that socioeconomic status and perceived adequacy of emotional support correlated positively with survival for people with localized cancers. For most cancers, incidence and prognosis was worse for those with fewer emotional supports, with socially isolated women and unmarried men at particularly elevated risk of dying from cancer. However, a different pattern was noted in one study of women with breast cancer (Ell et al., 1992). While perceived emotional support continued to be a protective factor, being married was a risk factor. The suggested explanation for this finding was the increased stress the disease created in the families and in the women themselves. Especially stressful was the necessity for these women to give up or radically change their usual roles in the family.

Aversive life events also may have a relationship to health. Sabbioni (1991) reported that students with high loneliness scores during school examination periods had signs of impaired cellular immunity while bereaved spouses showed decrements in immune system functioning as early as one month after the death of the spouse. Sabbioni also reported that women who experienced severe life events and difficulties during the postoperative disease-free interval after treatment for breast cancer were at increased risk for a recurrence.

In an early study, LeShan (1966) discovered a high incidence among cancer survivors of overwhelming early personal loss. LeShan also noted an association between later loss and cancer (Locke & Colligan, 1987). A common pattern that emerged from LeShan's interviews of 250 people who were diagnosed with cancer included a bleak and lonely childhood leading to a pessimistic view of the likelihood of achieving close and rewarding relationships. At some later point, many of these people found a job or another person they believed would be very rewarding to them and in whom they made a great investment only to lose that person or involvement less than a year before they were diagnosed with cancer. Although the prognostic implications of this information are unclear, the association is thought provoking.

A study of medical students yielded similar findings. Those who reported feeling emotionally distant from one or both parents had an unusually high incidence of death from cancer at follow-up thirty years later (Thomas, Dusynski, & Shaffer, 1979).

In a review of the literature, Watson and Ramirez (1991) observed that multiple studies found that major life stressors were unusually likely to have occurred within two years of the diagnosis of gastric cancer. A major loss was unusually likely to have been experienced within the five years before being diagnosed with lung cancer.

Major losses and other significant life experiences, like person-ality style, seem to be only one of many factors associated with the incidence and prognosis of cancer but they seem to have an addi-tive effect. According to Watson and Ramirez (1991, p. 67), "Stress-ful life experiences are not necessary for tumour growth nor are they sufficient by themselves to cause disease progression." However, they may play an important role for some subgroups, particularly people who suppress negative emotions and are prone to feelings of help-lessness and hopelessness.

Overview of Chapter

A substantial body of literature suggests a connection between psy-chological and physiological factors to the incidence and course of cancer. This does not mean that emotions cause cancer but rather that if there is susceptibility to cancer or exposure to carcinogens, the added impact of psychological factors may make a critical dif-ference (Moyers, 1993). This relationship seems particularly strong for cancers that are etiologically linked to hormonal factors (such as breast, ovarian, endometrial, and prostate cancers) or to the immune system (for example, leukemias, lymphomas) (Andersen,

Kiecolt-Glaser, & Glaser, 1994). This connection seems to be strongest for people in the middle adult years; in childhood cancer, genetics typically play a powerful role while in the elderly, the immune system commonly is weakened and may be less responsive. The relationship also seems particularly important for people who have been diagnosed with early-stage cancers (stage I or II). However, relationships also have been demonstrated between emotions and cancer for other types of cancer and for metastasized or advanced cancer as well.

Personal qualities associated with a good prognosis include the following:

- Fighting spirit

- Positive avoidance

- Strong, supportive relationships

- Ability to cope effectively and flexibly with stress

On the other hand, factors associated with a poor prognosis or a high incidence of cancer include the following:

- Fatalism

- Hopelessness and helplessness

- Anxiety and depression

- Suppression of emotions

- A lifestyle characterized by isolation, poor family relationships during childhood, low socioeconomic status, and major losses

Research also suggests that personal qualities associated with a good prognosis can be learned and developed while those associated with a poor prognosis can be minimized through psychotherapy. For people who have been diagnosed with cancer, that change can make an important difference in the course of the disease as well as in ability to cope with the diagnosis and its impact. The goal of this book is to help therapists develop the tools and understanding they need to help people strengthen those qualities that will help protect them from cancer as well as cope with the experience of having cancer.

Understanding the Cancer Survivor

The diagnosis of cancer is almost universally an extremely upsetting and difficult experience. Glanz and Lerman (1992) found that 80 percent of people diagnosed with cancer reported experiencing significant emotional distress.

However, people's reactions to the diagnosis and experience of having cancer vary enormously. Differences in reaction of course are to some extent determined by physiological dimensions, the nature and prognosis of the cancer as well as its physical effects. However, individual and interpersonal variables also have a profound impact on how people cope with cancer. The purpose of this chapter is to provide information on the nature of those variables. The Resources section at the back of this book includes a prototype for a series of counseling sessions with people diagnosed with cancer that illustrates the application of some of the material in this chapter. This information should help therapists assess the strength and nature of relevant personal variables and plan the therapy so it effectively addresses the person's needs and concerns. The material in this chapter also should help therapists focus on the whole person rather than the disease. As Remen put it (Moyers, 1993, p. 348), "Who you are is not somebody with cancer. Who you are is somebody. Somebody who matters."

Demographic Information

Before beginning an initial exploratory interview, therapists should obtain basic demographic information on the person. Because people with cancer typically begin psychotherapy with strong emotions barely held in check, collection of demographic information should take as little time as possible and might be gathered through a brief written intake questionnaire given to the person immediately before the first session or even at the end of that session if the person appears visibly upset from the outset. Since demographic variables such as gender, age, race, and ethnicity can have an impact on people's reactions to a diagnosis of cancer as well as to the treatment they receive, this information should be ascertained.

Age and Stage and Their Impact on Reactions to Cancer

Studies have found that younger people with cancer are more at risk for emotional distress (Andersen, 1992) and for the development of anticipatory nausea in response to chemotherapy (Payne, 1989). For them, cancer is usually unexpected. They may have little experience in dealing with serious illness, may have misconceptions about cancer, and may feel isolated and different from their peers because of the diagnosis. In addition, their physical appearance may have great importance for them and they may have looked forward to bearing children; cancer and its treatment may pose a threat to their self-image and their future goals.

Rose (1993) found that young adults (ages nineteen to forty) with cancer felt a particularly strong need to vent their emotions. They desired a high level of involvement in medical decisions affecting them and were likely to feel they did not receive as much support as they needed.

Older people, too, often have considerable difficulty coping with cancer but for different reasons. Their emotional and financial resources may be depleted, sometimes as a result of other illnesses, and they may be living alone or without caretakers to assist them. On the other hand, older women had less fear of a recurrence of cancer than did other age and gender groups, perhaps because they felt they already had completed most of their family-related goals (Glanz & Lerman, 1992). Rose (1993) found that older people (fifty-six to seventy-five) with cancer reported receiving less support than younger people with cancer but actually expressed greater satisfaction with their interactions with health care providers, suggesting they had lower expectations than other age groups.

In general, people in midlife, roughly between ages thirty-five and sixty-five, cope most effectively with cancer; they already have weathered many challenges in their lives, may have experience with serious illness, probably have a partner who can provide physical and emotional support, and are likely to have the financial resources they need to obtain good care. They have already begun to think in terms of time left and can imagine death as something that will happen to them (Schlossberg, 1984). They seem to require the least amount of outside support because they have their own support systems and usually are satisfied with the support they receive. The similarity in age between health care providers and adults in midlife also may facilitate communication and provision of appropriate support (Rose, 1993).

Age is related to psychosocial stages of development and these too are important to consider when assessing the impact of cancer. The disease may interfere with successful progression through age-appropriate tasks and milestones. The adolescent with cancer, for example, may have particular difficulty developing a positive sense of identity and independence (Ettinger & Heiney, 1993). People in their twenties may have difficulty with the threat cancer treatment may pose to their ability to reproduce while those in their thirties may have particularly strong concerns around sexuality (Oktay & Walter, 1991).

Many models exist that delineate the stages of human development and that may provide information on the stage- and age-related impact of cancer. Probably the best known of these is Erikson's (1963) classic eight-stage model:

1. Basic trust versus basic mistrust

2. Autonomy versus shame and doubt

3. Initiative versus guilt

4. Industry versus inferiority

5. Identity versus role confusion

6. Intimacy versus isolation

7. Generativity versus stagnation

8. Ego integrity versus despair

The first two represent the psychosocial stages of infancy; cancer in a very young child usually is terrifying to a family and may raise issues related to blame, communication, the child's future, loss, and the integrity of the family (Doka, 1993). Cancer diagnosed during the next two stages, those of childhood, is likely to lead to concerns around growth, independence, autonomy, and differentness. Stage five is typically negotiated during adolescence; a diagnosis of cancer during that stage may raise questions of identity, peer relations, intimacy, and separation. During stage six, young adulthood, issues of family, relationships, careers, insurance, and procreation are likely to accompany a diagnosis of cancer. Stage seven usually occurs during middle adulthood; cancer during those years may raise awareness of mortality as well as issues related to career, family, finances, and the meaning of one's life. Finally, cancer diagnosed during stage eight, the later years, while still a shock, may lead to a life review of goals, accomplishments, and disappointments.

Schlossberg (1984) observed that of course not all people of approximately the same age have the same developmental needs and tasks. She suggested considering time from three perspectives: historical or calendar time, life time or chronological age, and socially defined time. All three of these have an impact on age reactions to cancer.

For example, a thirty-five-year-old woman with two children, ages five and seven, a professional career, and a diagnosis of breast cancer in 1995 will have many issues related to age and stage. Few of her peers will have had personal experience with cancer and so she may feel different and isolated. She may fear the impact her diagnosis and possible death will have on her young children. Concerns about physical appearance and sexuality are likely to be important. Her already demanding schedule, and the common expectation that women of this era should be able to manage career and family, probably will compound her resistance to prolonged and perhaps incapacitating treatments. All of these issues should be considered by therapists working with such a client.

Age and stage interact with other variables to determine a person's reaction to cancer. For example, research has found that single people have higher death rates from cancer, especially if they are older and are part of a lower socioeconomic group (Andersen, 1992). This pattern probably can be explained by multiple factors including inadequate medical care, personal neglect, lack of information on resources, limited support systems, finances, and personality factors.

A study of the amount of social services provided to cancer survivors and their families indicated that the groups using the most services included women who were younger and who did not have a child living at home and people who were separated or divorced (Royse & Dhooper, 1988). Other groups identified as having a high need for services were the elderly, people who were widowed, and single parents. Evidently, the interaction of several demographic variables affects cancer-related needs as well as response to the disease.

Ethnicity and Culture and Their Impact on Reactions to Cancer

Ethnicity and culture, too, have an impact on people's reactions to a diagnosis of cancer. Ethnic and cultural background can of course influence genetics, resources, ability to negotiate the health care system, and health habits. Moyers (1993), for example, reported that fewer medical tests are performed on women and on men of color. These factors can in turn affect incidence and prognosis of cancer.

Ethnicity and cultural context can also exert an indirect influence on prognosis through culturally mediated attitudes toward life, illness, treatment, and death as well as ways people express and cope with pain, suffering, and grief. For people with a Japanese heritage, cancer commonly is equated with death; those with Irish roots typically accept pain and suffering with stoic resignation; while people with a Jewish background are much more likely to aggressively explore all sources of treatment (Rosen, 1990). Many people from Asian backgrounds view surgery as mutilation and may refuse surgery and even fear having blood drawn for that reason (Gon, 1993). I have found that some women from Asian backgrounds need particular help in communicating assertively with male physicians and in developing a fighting spirit while people with Middle Eastern ancestry have little difficulty rallying family support and expressing their needs to physicians but are reluctant to become involved in support groups. Exploration of people's ethnic backgrounds and culturally derived beliefs can promote understanding of their responses to the diagnosis and treatment of cancer and can guide the development of appropriate treatment plans.

Gender and Its Impact on Reactions to Cancer

Gender is another important variable in determining response to cancer. Although men and women seem to be equally distressed at the diagnosis, they tend to use different coping mechanisms (Fife, Kennedy, & Robinson, 1994). Men have been found to make significantly greater use of avoidance and distancing than women while women coping with cancer are more likely to use positive and active coping strategies and to seek social and religious support. Although women seem more adept at using family support than men, they tend not to use professional resources as well as men. In general, men coping with cancer focus on solving concrete problems presented by the disease while women focus on modifying their emotional reactions and typically make a more positive adjustment to the diagnosis of cancer.

The Family Context

The demographic factors of age, ethnicity, and gender are only a beginning in understanding people with cancer. They also should be viewed in terms of their context. Probably the most important context to consider is the family (used in its broadest sense here to refer to functional as well as biological family). According to Rolland (1994, p. 1), "The impact of a diagnosis of cancer or daily living with a serious disability reverberates throughout the family system, leaving no one untouched."

Rolland (1994) wrote of the importance of establishing a functional family-illness system, in which the family has a shared and articulated understanding of the nature and demands of the illness, of themselves as a functional unit, of the family's development, and of their values and belief systems. To facilitate establishment of such a system, therapists are encouraged to evaluate the following domains of family functioning:

1.   The composition and structure of the family: Who the important family members are, the nature of the family constellation, the family hierarchy, the level of cohesion in the family, subsystems, boundaries, and levels of adaptability and flexibility

2.   The developmental stage of the nuclear family: For example, newly married, launching adult children, retirement

3.   Family dynamics and communication: Patterns of interaction and communication within the family, alliances and conflicts, constraints on communication, usual roles and responsibilities in the family

4.   The family circumstances: Strengths and weaknesses of the family prior to the diagnosis, nature and impact of other stressors, financial and emotional resources

5.   Important family background information: Previous losses and disappointments, ways of dealing with past stressors, experience with illness and death

6.   Family response to cancer: Individual and group meanings attributed to the disease, attributions of its cause, expected outcome

The following sections provide additional information on the relationship between family context and reactions to cancer.

The Composition and Structure of the Family

The experience of cancer can change a family. The illness itself as well as the medical team may become like additional members of the family and the family needs to expand its boundaries enough to make this possible. Families often become more cohesive when faced with serious illness, and this may offer them necessary strength and support as long as it does not prevent them from benefiting from outside support systems. Similarly, families with religious or spiritual beliefs may benefit from greater involvement with their religion as long as their belief system is flexible and does not lead them toward self-blame or extreme denial.

For most people with cancer, being married or being in a committed relationship has a protective function. Kiecolt-Glaser et al. (1984) compared women who were married with those who were separated or divorced. They found that the married women had the best immune system functioning, with those who reported being happily married having the best immune system functioning of the group.

Unfortunately, being part of a family does not always have a positive impact on cancer survivors. Families may resent the disease as well as the ill person, particularly if significant changes in roles and family functioning and unwelcome alliances are necessitated by the disease.

The impact of the disease is likely to be particularly devastating if it causes a change in the marital relationship and in the family hierarchy. For example, in the Lewis family, consisting of parents and two sons, the mother had been the strongest force in the family; she had strong alliances with both her sons and a weak alliance with her husband. When she was diagnosed with cancer, she was forced to yield her role in the family to her husband who then withdrew further from his wife and bonded more with his sons. The mother felt she had lost not only her role in the family but her relationships with her sons and her husband while the sons suffered from the loss of the mother they had known. Both sons and the mother sought counseling because of depression.

Family roles, as well as expectations, often are linked to gender stereotypes. In a traditional family, the husband may be expected to be the breadwinner while the wife's primary role is to bear and raise the children. Cancer may interfere with childbearing as well as with employment. While such an impact will be difficult for almost all families, it may be especially difficult for families that have narrowly defined gender roles. Conflicts around priorities related to gender roles may be especially difficult to handle; the young married woman with children may become angry and resentful when she is expected to care for her widowed father with cancer while her brothers are not expected to help.

The Developmental Stage of the Nuclear Family

Carter and McGoldrick (1988, p. 13) identified what they call "the stages of the intact middle-class American family life cycle" that delineate six stages of family development and their accompanying transitions and issues. The model encompasses the following stages:

1. *Leaving home:* Single young adults—achieving emotional and financial responsibility for oneself
2. *The joining of families through marriage:* The new couple—forming and making a commitment to a new system, realigning former relationships to include the spouse
3. *Families with young children:* Adjusting the marital system and other family relationships to accommodate children; collaborating on childrearing, finances, and household responsibilities
4. *Families with adolescents:* Increasing flexibility in family boundaries to allow adolescents' independence, caring for grandparents, and increased focus on midlife marital and career issues
5. *Launching children and moving on:* Accepting many exits and entrances into the family system; redefining relationships with spouse, adult children, parents, in-laws, grandchildren
6. *Families in later life:* Accommodating the shift in generational roles, maintaining relationships and a satisfying lifestyle in the face of physical decline, dealing with loss, life review, and integration

Using this model to assess the stage of a given family's development can be helpful in two ways. If the family is following a pattern that is reflected in this model, therapists can use the model to promote understanding for themselves and their clients of the impact cancer is likely to have on the family. The diagnosis of cancer often impairs normal family development and functioning, at least temporarily, and areas likely to be most affected can be identified by the model. A family in an unstable or transitional stage, involving departures from the nuclear family, may have particular difficulty coping with cancer.

If a family is following a pattern that does not match the model, perhaps marrying and bearing children in midlife, they may have particular trouble coping with a diagnosis of cancer. They may already feel isolated because most of their age peers have very different concerns and family patterns and the family may have fewer support systems as a result. If cancer itself seems to be particularly untimely, perhaps striking a child or an adult with young children, that can compound even further the sense of differentness and isolation.

Family Dynamics and Communication

Families will communicate about cancer as they have communicated about other issues. Families that prohibit expression of emotion as well as discussion of difficult or upsetting topics seem to have particular difficulty dealing with cancer. Fears and misconceptions mount, with no opportunity to dispel them.

Therapists should pay attention to the styles of communication (for example, verbal, behavioral), the channels of communication, and the family messages about what discussion is permitted. By building on the strongest available means of communication, perhaps through the healthiest family member, or by using writing or family activities as a mode of communication, efforts can be made to increase openness and self-expression in the family system.

Family Circumstances

Other stressors and crises, concurrent with the diagnosis of cancer, can increase the difficulty the family faces in coping with cancer. Families who are struggling with other major stressors, particularly those involving loss and illness, may have depleted resources and may need considerable help in dealing with cancer.

For most families, maintaining the elements and patterns of their lives that were important before the diagnosis of cancer is reassuring and helps them to avoid excessive focusing on the disease. Family rituals and celebrations can be especially helpful in communicating the message that life will go on. This can be challenging; one woman who was undergoing chemotherapy wanted to attend an out-of-town wedding on the weekend she expected to lose her hair. Because she recognized the importance to her and her family of her presence at the wedding, she had her hair done and her wig prepared at the same time to deal with all possibilities.

Coping with cancer may be facilitated by using outside resources such as friends who will care for the children, a relative who will prepare meals, colleagues who will provide transportation to treatments, or a cleaning service to keep the house in order. People who are affiliated with a church or synagogue may receive emotional as well as practical help from their clergy and associated support services such as church caring committees. These support systems can reduce the pressure on the family, free them to focus attention on coping with cancer, and maintain the homeostasis of the family. A review of the family's current situation should include identification of potential outside resources and a discussion of the use the family generally has made of such resources, facilitating encouragement of even greater use of these sources of help during the present crisis.

Although nearly all families will be changed by living with cancer, change often seems to be in the direction the family has been moving. The family that already is fragmented and contentious may reach a crossroads that will precipitate a divorce while the family that is supportive and positive may find that coping with cancer increases mutual appreciation and commitment.

Important Family Background Information

Rosen (1990, p. 8), discussing families facing death, wrote, "Family is not merely an assemblage of individuals; it is those same individuals inextricably intertwined in ways that are constantly interactive and mutually reinforcing. And family, in the fullest sense of the word, embraces all generations—past, present, and future—those living, those dead, and those yet to be born." Rosen's words apply equally to families facing serious illness. The family history, its culture, its beliefs, all will affect the efforts of the present family to cope with cancer and will in turn shape the responses of future generations to similar concerns.

Family Response to Cancer

Families affected by cancer seem to formulate both group and individual understandings of the cause of the disease, its outcome, and the best way to address it. This process seems to be a natural reaction to an unexpected and unwanted event and can help people accept and make sense of the diagnosis. Families may lean toward a biological explanation (your mother had cancer and you inherited the cancer gene from her) or one of personal responsibility (you have cancer because you eat too much junk food). They may feel optimistic (the doctor says the prognosis is good; we just have to get through this) or pessimistic (I'll have to raise the children alone, I just know it). They may be solicitous and supportive, taking on many of the responsibilities of the cancer survivor, or they may believe that the best way to deal with cancer is to think about it as little as possible and to go on with business as usual.

Reactions of family members of cancer survivors can be as varied as those of the survivors themselves and can be compounded by individual differences within the family. Consequently, in addition to determining family beliefs about the cause, prognosis, and appropriate response to cancer, therapists should look at both unified family messages and individual belief systems, paying particular attention to the congruence between the beliefs and needs of cancer survivors and their family members. Communication and support can be undermined when, for example, the wife believes, "I'm going to die; we need to make plans for the children's care" and the husband believes, "My wife will be fine; she just shouldn't think so much about cancer."

Also potentially harmful to the family as well as the cancer survivor are meanings attributed to the disease that increase guilt and hopelessness. Common negative explanations include punishment for misdeeds, blaming others, injustice, genetics, negligence and poor health habits, and bad luck. Donald, for example, believed that cancer was his punishment from God for changing his religious affiliation when he married. People and families with rigid and extreme beliefs about control, responsibility, and religion seem particularly prone to negative beliefs such as these.

Lerner (Moyers, 1993, p. 337) has taken a strong stance on the unfortunate tendency for people to blame themselves for developing cancer: "One of the illnesses of the 'new age' is the view, 'I caused my cancer, I should be able to reverse it.' That's an incredibly simplistic and unfortunate attitude. We live in an age where cancer is essentially an epidemic illness. . . . It may be that psychological factors in an individual life contributed to the multifactorial mix that caused the emergence of a cancer, but to say that you caused your illness because of some set of events or some way that you related to the world ignores all the other things over which you had absolutely no control." Therapists need to be especially careful to address issues of self-blame and, in seeking to empower their clients, to avoid attributing blame for the cancer to the person.

Rolland (1994) stressed the importance of helping people create a meaning for their disease that promotes competence and mastery. By exploring beliefs on health; human nature; religion; family, friends, and other support systems; mind-body relationships; responsibility; and illness and its causes, therapists can lay the foundation for helping people make sense of cancer in a way that empowers them and gives them hope.

Using Genograms in Family Assessment

Genograms are a useful and powerful tool in family therapy (McGoldrick & Gerson, 1985). Genograms typically diagram at least three generations of a family, providing identifying and demographic information (dates of births and deaths, religion, ethnicity, occupations, marriages, divorces), indications of patterns of family relationships, important family events, and any other information relevant to the purpose of a particular genogram. Discussion of the genogram can then facilitate understanding of multigenerational patterns and messages that are having an impact on the present family.

In developing a genogram with families coping with cancer, the therapist would pay particular attention to listing causes of death and the incidence of serious illness. Discussion then could explore what is recalled about the experience of each illness and death, their impact on the individual and the family, whether and how people were informed of illnesses and deaths, recurrent types of illness in the family, how the illnesses were handled in the family, and impressions the present family members have of the circumstances of the illnesses and deaths. An example of such a genogram appears in Figure 2.1.

The genogram illustrates the family of Margo, a forty-six-year-old woman dealing with a diagnosis of breast cancer. Her mother and her maternal grandmother after whom she was named died in midlife of breast cancer while her paternal grandmother and an aunt died of colon cancer. Another aunt had breast cancer but is still alive. Her father, on the other hand, died of a heart attack when he was eighty-four. Most of the men in her family died suddenly without suffering, as her father did. The women, on the other hand, suffered greatly from cancer and its treatments.

Although Margo had never been close to her mother, she vividly recalled her mother experiencing an agonizing death: "She died like a dog." At the time of Margo's mother's illness, limitations in medical knowledge, prevailing secrecy and stigma surrounding a diagnosis of cancer, and norms of stoicism and extreme privacy in Margo's family of origin prevented her mother from asking for and receiving the medical and emotional help that Margo felt her mother needed. Margo herself felt considerable guilt at her reactions; as an adolescent, she was frightened and repelled by her mother's illness and resulting surgery and withdrew from her mother during the illness.

Now Margo was herself a woman with breast cancer with an adolescent daughter. In her mind, cancer was a sentence to a

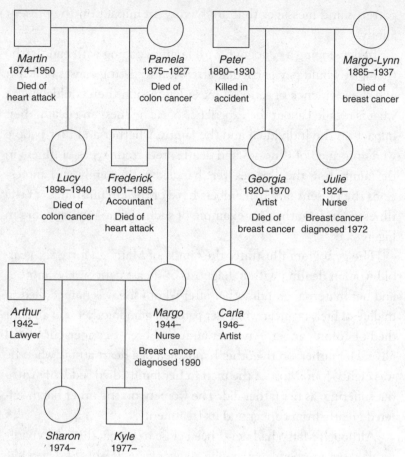

Figure 2.1. Genogram of Margo's Family.

certain, untimely, and dreadful death unlike her very different experience with her father's death from a sudden heart attack after a long and rewarding life. At the time she sought therapy, Margo's heightened anxiety was interfering with her treatment ("What's the point of having chemotherapy? I'm going to die anyway") and was exacerbating the worry and sense of helplessness her immediate family members were experiencing. Her younger sister, usually a strong source of support for Margo, had become withdrawn and distant, perhaps out of fear that she would be the next member of the family to develop breast cancer. By exploring the antecedents of

Margo's anxieties through the genogram, she was able to get a clearer picture of her disease and her reactions and to see the differences between her situation and that of her mother in terms of both prognosis and available treatments.

Margo is part of a growing group of people who have seen parents, siblings, and others close to them deal with cancer and its difficult treatments and sometimes die from the disease. According to Holland (1992), these people are particularly likely to feel great anxiety in response to a diagnosis of cancer and to have difficulty with medical tests and treatments as well as self-diagnostic procedures.

However, a history of coping with cancer can also have a positive impact and this too can be elicited through the genogram. Robin and her husband David, for example, had successfully dealt with David's diagnosis of testicular cancer many years earlier. Now that Robin was diagnosed with colon cancer, they were optimistic that once again the outcome would be positive and they diligently gathered information and medical opinions to make the best possible decisions about Robin's treatment.

Although direct past experience with cancer is likely to exert a particularly strong impact on people coping with cancer, the genogram also provides a useful vehicle for considering other relevant family background factors discussed earlier in this chapter such as generational patterns of family roles and responsibilities, ethnic and cultural messages, gender stereotypes, and family stages.

Individual Dynamics and Cancer

Dynamics and issues within the person diagnosed with cancer affect coping abilities just as do dynamics and issues within the family. Aspects of the person that are important to consider include the following:

- Psychological resources, quality of life, and response to the diagnosis

- Physical health and medical history

- Cognitive style

- Social networks, interpersonal skills, and relationships

- Career and work history, financial resources

- Spiritual beliefs, sense of purpose, religious practices

- Symptoms and prognosis c ͭ the disease

Psychological Resources and Responses

Holland (1992, p. 108) defined quality of life for people with can-cer as "the level of patients' functioning in the psychological, social, physical, work, and sexual domains of their lives." These domains encompass the resources that will mediate the emotional impact of cancer on the person. Becoming aware of the cancer survivor's needs and resources, both before and after cancer, is essential to understanding and helping that person.

Although many people have the resources to cope successfully with cancer, others do not. According to Moorey and Greer (1989, p. viii), "It has become apparent that many cancer patients, although adequately treated physically, develop severe emotional and psychological problems which are inadequately managed and, at times, not even recognized." Common emotional difficulties include depression, anxiety, guilt, feelings of worthlessness, anger, and suicidal ideation.

Some studies indicate that nearly one half of cancer patients have a mental disorder according to the criteria in the *Diagnostic and Statistical Manual of Mental Disorders* (American Psychiatric Association, 1994). One study of both hospitalized and ambulatory cancer patients found that 47 percent met the criteria for a mental disorder; 68 percent of those had adjustment disorders with depressed or anxious mood, 13 percent had major depressive disor-ders, 8 percent had cognitive mental disorders, 7 percent had personality disorders, and 4 percent had anxiety disorders. Nearly 90 percent of those disorders developed in response to the diagnosis, symptoms, and treatment of cancer (Massie & Holland, 1992). Another study of people who were hospitalized for treatment of cancer found that 66 percent were depressed, 24 percent of them severely depressed (Bukberg, Penman, & Holland, 1984). This is a much higher incidence than in the general population, where depression has been found in 6 percent (Andersen, 1992). At highest risk for the development of mental disorders in reaction to cancer are people with a history of mood disorders, substance use disorders, or concurrent illnesses that cause depressive symptoms; people with unresolved grief; and people experiencing poorly controlled pain as well as those in the advanced stages of cancer (Massie & Holland, 1990; Vachon, 1987). These factors, along with previous suicide attempts, a family history of suicide, recent bereavements, and few social supports, are associated with an increased risk of cancer-related suicide (Massie & Holland, 1992). Although fewer than 2 percent of people with cancer commit suicide, the risk is higher than for the general population and suicidal thinking seems to be very common among people with cancer (Breitbart, 1989).

In addition to determining whether emotional disorders or symptoms are present, clinicians should assess people's methods of coping. This can be accomplished by exploring their ways of handling previous stressful circumstances and approaches they plan to use in dealing with cancer. The previous chapter reviewed the relationship of coping style to both medical prognosis and emotional adjustment and identified five salient coping styles in cancer survivors: fighting spirit, avoidance or denial, fatalism, helplessness/hopelessness, and anxious preoccupation. Understanding these approaches to coping with cancer can facilitate assessment of a particular person's style.

Coping styles and degree of pathology are only two aspects that can be assessed by therapists seeking to understand the cancer survivor. Other aspects include self-image and self-esteem, lifestyle and quality of life, underlying personality style, level of adjustment prior to the diagnosis of cancer, and any other personal variables that seem relevant to the clinician or the cancer survivor.

Physical Health and Medical History

The physical health of cancer survivors, particularly their experience of pain, body changes, and aversive side effects of treatment, have an impact on how they cope with cancer. In addition, their previous experiences in dealing with cancer and other serious illnesses will color their reactions to the present illness. Jevne (1990) found that having had a family member, friend, or significant other who had cancer compounded the challenge presented by cancer. Those people with previous cancer experience were more likely than those without such an experience to manifest severe marital problems and anxiety after their own diagnosis of cancer. Exploration of both present health and previous experience with illnesses in the survivor and significant others offers another useful source of information on a person's response to cancer.

Cognitive Style

A diagnosis of cancer usually requires cancer survivors to assemble information and opinions and make decisions that will affect the rest of their lives. Some cancer survivors put their fate into the hands of the first physician they see and allow that person to direct their medical treatment. At the other extreme, some cancer survivors obtain multiple opinions and review the medical literature on their conditions in an effort to determine the treatment that is most likely to be effective. The extent of a person's information gathering depends on many factors, including intellectual level, educational background and familiarity with library research, level of anxiety and confusion, usual style of addressing problems, and the medical and informational resources readily available to them.

Although obtaining substantial knowledge about their disease and its treatment may be empowering and helpful to many cancer survivors, others feel overwhelmed and frightened by extensive information. This is another important dimension to consider that will contribute to clinicians' overall understanding of their clients who are cancer survivors.

Social Networks, Skills, and Relationships

Social support has been found to be associated with improved adjustment, emotional well-being, and reduced fear of recurrence in cancer survivors (Glanz & Lerman, 1992). What is most important is not the quantity of cancer survivors' social supports but rather their *perceived* quality (Winefield & Neuling, 1987). As Ornish (Moyers, 1993, p. 105) put it, "Anything that promotes a sense of intimacy, community, and connection can be healing."

Unfortunately, many cancer survivors are reluctant to discuss their fears and feelings with friends and family; they may not want to upset the people they care about, they may feel guilt or shame connected to their disease, or they may have weak communication skills and a personal style that prevents sharing strong feelings and experiences. This arena too warrants assessment in order to understand cancer survivors' reactions, resources, and treatment needs.

Career and Work History, Financial Resources

Having rewarding employment that provides sick pay as well as adequate financial resources, including medical insurance, disability insurance, and life insurance, can help to allay some of the fears surrounding a diagnosis of cancer. People who have secure employment to which they are eager to return, as well as the financial resources they need for their cancer treatments and for the care of themselves and their families, usually will find it easier to devote their full attention to getting well.

Spiritual Beliefs and Sense of Purpose

A sense of meaning or purpose to one's life as well as strong spiritual beliefs can contribute greatly to a person's efforts to deal with a diagnosis of cancer. Mullen, Smith, and Hill (1993) defined a sense of *coherence* as the belief that stimuli are structured, predictable, and make sense; that resources are available to meet the demands of these stimuli; and that these demands are challenges that merit investment of effort and involvement. They found that people who had a sense of coherence about their disease were less likely to experience high stress than people who did not have this sense of coherence. Spiritual resources and family strengths offer pathways to achieving this sense of coherence.

Nearly all people with cancer experience a sort of existential plight, in which the world they know and their very existence is threatened (Lynn, 1986). For some, this phase is transient and only mildly troubling while for others it is a turning point, potentially creating or intensifying serious psychosocial problems.

Spiritual beliefs, which may or may not be reflected in involvement in traditional religion, may help people cope with the existential plight and upheaval that often accompanies a diagnosis of cancer. Faith in a higher power may moderate fears and give a sense of hope and help, while involvement in a religious or spiritual community may provide much needed support systems. On the other hand, perceived injustice in a diagnosis of cancer, particularly in a young person, may raise religious doubts and may lead people to turn away from their usual place of worship. Exploration of spiritual beliefs and practices held both before and subsequent to the diagnosis of cancer is another important approach to understanding cancer survivors and their resources.

Symptoms and Prognosis of the Disease

Finally, it is important to obtain information on the symptoms of the disease and its treatment as well as the prognosis of the disease. This may involve acquiring a release of information and communicating with the person's physician. Cancer is, understandably, especially difficult to handle if it causes pain and disfigurement and if the prognosis is negative or uncertain. Both survivor and therapist should be as clear as possible about the likely course and impact of the disease as they proceed with their work together.

Overview of Chapter

Taking a holistic approach to understanding people with cancer is essential to treating them effectively. There are many factors in cancer survivors and their families that may affect their reactions to the diagnosis and treatment of their disease as well as their emotional needs. Only by considering personal and interpersonal dimensions and dynamics of cancer survivors can therapists determine their needs and resources and plan treatment strategies that have a high likelihood of success.

3

· ·

Using Standardized Assessment

Chapter Two of this book provided some guidelines for gathering information on cancer survivors via interviews and other nonstandardized approaches. Although these approaches often will provide sufficient understanding of the person, sometimes the style of the therapist, the nature of the client, or the treatment plan indicates the use of a more structured approach to assessment.

Reasons for Using Standardized Assessment

The use of standardized inventories with cancer survivors can accomplish several goals: provide a baseline measurement of symptoms that will help both therapists and clients to assess progress; indicate whether severe pathology is present, perhaps necessitating a referral for medication or hospitalization; and give therapists greater understanding of the person, thereby facilitating treatment planning and communication of empathy and support.

At the same time, therapists should avoid overemphasizing testing with cancer survivors. Therapy should generally focus on mutual discussion of troubling issues related to the disease. That discussion will usually serve as the primary vehicle for assessment. Testing should be used cautiously because of its potential association with medical tests and procedures and the possibility that it may detract from the development of a positive therapeutic relationship. Cancer survivors have already experienced extensive, painful, and probably dehumanizing medical tests and procedures, and psychotherapy should seek to counteract those experiences with warmth, support, and concern.

Mental Disorders in Cancer Survivors

Cancer survivors may be free of mental disorders, they may have preexisting mental disorders that are likely to be exacerbated by the stress of coping with cancer, or they may have mental disorders that developed in response to the diagnosis of cancer. In order to provide the best possible treatment, clinicians need to determine whether a client does have a mental disorder, the nature of that disorder, and whether that disorder resulted from or was affected by the diagnosis of cancer.

Diagnostic and Statistical Manual of Mental Disorders

In the United States, as well as in many other countries, the criteria for determining the presence of mental disorders are provided by the fourth edition of the *Diagnostic and Statistical Manual of Mental Disorders (DSM-IV)* (American Psychiatric Association, 1994). Three disorders in that manual are particularly likely to result from the diagnosis of cancer: Adjustment Disorder, Major Depressive Disorder, and Generalized Anxiety Disorder or Anxiety Disorder Not Otherwise Specified. Barraclough (1994) reported that 30 percent of people with cancer meet the *DSM* criteria for an Adjustment Disorder while 20 percent meet the criteria for other disorders, usually depressive or anxiety disorders. In addition, preexisting conditions such as substance use disorders and personality disorders may also be prevalent in cancer survivors and may be exacerbated by dealing with cancer.

Adjustment Disorders

According to the *DSM-IV*, Adjustment Disorders involve "the development of emotional or behavioral symptoms in response to an identifiable stressor occurring within three months of the onset of the stressor" and are characterized either by "marked distress that is in excess of what would be expected from exposure to the stressor" or "significant impairment in social or occupational functioning" (American Psychiatric Association, 1994, p. 626). The maximum duration of an Adjustment Disorder is six months beyond the termination of the stressor or its consequences; for people coping with cancer, this would mean six months beyond the end of treatments for the disease. Six types of Adjustment Disorders have been identified: Adjustment Disorders with Depressed Mood, with Anxiety, with Mixed Anxiety and Depressed Mood, with Disturbance of Conduct, with Mixed Disturbance of Emotions and Conduct, and Unspecified (for example, physical complaints, social withdrawal, work inhibition). Adults who are coping with cancer are most likely to manifest symptoms of anxiety and depression while children are more likely to demonstrate behavioral difficulties as well as anxiety and depression. Cancer survivors, as well as their caregivers, may be diagnosed with an Adjustment Disorder if they manifest some relatively mild but clinically significant affective or behavioral disturbance in response to dealing with cancer. Although these symptoms certainly need to be addressed in therapy, Adjustment Disorders typically have an excellent prognosis and usually do not require medication or hospitalization (Seligman, 1990a).

Major Depressive Disorders

More severe than an Adjustment Disorder is a Major Depressive Disorder. According to the *DSM-IV* (American Psychiatric Association, 1994), a Major Depressive Disorder has a minimum duration of two weeks and is characterized by at least five of the following symptoms, including at least one of the first two: feeling depressed most of the time, reduced interest or pleasure in activities, weight loss, sleep disturbance, psychomotor agitation or retardation, loss of energy, feelings of worthlessness or excessive guilt, impairment in thinking and decision making, and recurrent thoughts of death or suicide. In children, irritability often masks depression but is a common symptom of a Major Depressive Disorder.

Cancer survivors who are experiencing a Major Depressive Disorder seem particularly likely to have excessive guilt, blaming themselves for their disease; to be troubled by thoughts of death; and to feel immobilized in the face of the many decisions that usually must be made following the diagnosis of cancer. Symptoms such as eating and sleeping disturbances also may be present but are less reliable indicators of depression since they also may be caused by cancer treatments. Significant depression is particularly likely in people with advanced pancreatic cancer and in people with a first recurrence of their disease, but studies have found depression in 4.5 percent to 58 percent of all people with cancer (Hughes, 1987; Massie & Holland, 1990). Antidepressant medication is sometimes necessary, along with psychotherapy, for people with Major Depressive Disorders. In psychotherapy, emphasis on cognitive-behavioral interventions is likely to be more helpful in alleviating depressive symptoms than are supportive or affective interventions.

Anxiety Disorders

Anxiety is another prevalent symptom among cancer survivors. A Generalized Anxiety Disorder is typified by at least six months of excessive anxiety and worry about several aspects of one's life. People with this disorder also manifest at least three physiological signs of anxiety such as restlessness, fatigue, difficulty concentrating, irritability, muscle tension, and sleep disturbance.

Although cancer survivors may well present with the symptoms of a Generalized Anxiety Disorder, they seem even more likely to have an Anxiety Disorder Not Otherwise Specified. That disorder too is characterized primarily by excessive and uncontrollable anxiety but may have a briefer duration than the six-month minimum duration for a Generalized Anxiety Disorder and may include a mixture of anxiety and depressive symptoms. Phobic symptoms too may be present in an Anxiety Disorder Not Otherwise Specified; phobias focused on venipuncture, chemotherapy, and other procedures are not unusual in people undergoing treatment for cancer.

Cancer survivors experiencing anxiety disorders typically worry not only about their health but also about finances, family relationships, and their work. They feel tense and apprehensive, fearing that more bad news is imminent. Cognitive-behavioral interventions are effective with anxiety disorders as they are in treating depressive disorders (Seligman, 1990a). Relaxation techniques also are an important component of treating people with anxiety disorders.

Cognitive Mental Disorders

Older people with cancer, as well as those with advanced disease, metabolic and endocrine disturbances, brain lesions, and those receiving heavy doses of narcotics or steroids, are at particular risk of developing a cognitive mental disorder (Fleishman, Lesko, & Breitbart, 1993). Deliria is especially prevalent, found in 8 to 40 percent of people with cancer. Common early symptoms of deliria include changes in sleep patterns, restlessness, periods of disorientation, irritability, anger, withdrawal, and forgetfulness. Medication, as well as quiet and safe surroundings, stabilization, and one-to-one companionship, can reduce cognitive symptoms.

Common Preexisting Conditions

Little research has looked at preexisting conditions in cancer survivors. However, several disorders are likely to be common as preexisting conditions because of their association with cancer or with the personality patterns that have been found to be prevalent in cancer survivors (Temoshok & Dreher, 1992).

Several types of cancer are associated with the use of tobacco and alcohol. Consequently, people with such cancers as lung cancer or cancer of the mouth also may have a substance use disorder such as Alcohol Dependence, Alcohol Abuse, or Nicotine Dependence. Feelings of guilt and self-blame are particularly likely for people whose cancers bear a strong relationship to their behaviors. Although the diagnosis of cancer may lead some people to reduce behaviors that are associated with that disease, others actually may increase those behaviors because they reduce stress. Therapists dealing with people with substance use disorders must guard against increasing self-blame and recriminations in their clients; at the same time, behavioral interventions are indicated to help people reduce their self-destructive use of alcohol, cigarettes, and other substances.

Several personality disorders also seem likely to be common among cancer survivors. Personality disorders are characterized by long-standing, deeply ingrained, and pervasive impairment. Although people with personality disorders may achieve an adequate level of functioning and may never seek psychotherapy for their mental disorders, they will manifest impairment in at least two of the following areas: cognition, affect, interpersonal functioning, and impulse control (American Psychiatric Association, 1994). The following personality disorders seem most likely to be diagnosed in cancer survivors because of their relationship to what Temoshok and Dreher (1992) called the Type C or cancer-prone personality:

- *Schizoid Personality Disorder,* characterized primarily by difficulty expressing emotions, social isolation, and inadequate ability to cope effectively with stress

- *Avoidant Personality Disorder,* characterized primarily by social inhibition, feelings of inadequacy, and difficulty in self-expression

- *Dependent Personality Disorder,* characterized primarily by excessive reliance on others, feelings of helplessness, difficulty with self-expression, and lack of self-confidence

- *Obsessive-Compulsive Personality Disorder*, characterized primarily by perfectionism, inflexibility, and minimal involvement in social and leisure activities

Psychotherapy focused on helping people cope with cancer is likely to be more difficult if the person has a personality disorder. Typically, people with these disorders have poor insight, difficulty expressing their emotions, and difficulty making good use of support systems. Cancer survivors with personality disorders may require long-term therapy since the personality disorder may complicate efforts to help them cope with cancer.

Comprehensive Personality Inventories

Several personality inventories are available that provide a comprehensive picture of a person as well as information on the *DSM* diagnoses and appropriate treatment approaches. The best known of these are the Minnesota Multiphasic Personality Inventory and the Millon Clinical Multiaxial Inventory, both distributed by National Computer Systems, Minneapolis, Minnesota. These true-false, paper-pencil, computer-scored inventories are designed to assess the presence of psychopathology in older adolescents and adults. Both may be useful in helping clinicians determine whether and what mental disorders are present in a cancer survivor who seems unusually troubled or dysfunctional.

Assessment of Transient Psychological Symptoms

Regardless of whether a mental disorder is present in a cancer survivor, therapists may want to assess the presence and degree of symptoms as both a guide for treatment planning and a marker to assess progress. Several useful inventories are available that would meet these goals.

Profile of Mood States

The inventory that has been most widely used to assess transient symptoms in cancer survivors, as well as to determine how their quality of life can be improved, is the Profile of Mood States (POMS), distributed by EdITS, San Diego, California (McNair, Lorr, & Droppleman, 1992). The POMS consists of sixty-five rating scales on which respondents indicate the extent to which they have experienced specified feelings during the past week. The rating scales range from 0/not at all to 4/extremely and yield scores on the following six mood states: Tension-Anxiety, Depression-Dejection, Anger-Hostility, Vigor-Activity, Fatigue-Inertia, and Confusion-Bewilderment. A Total Mood Disturbance score can also be obtained from the POMS. Research has indicated that the POMS has good reliability and validity.

Use of the POMS with cancer survivors has shown that "cancer affects mood states and POMS profiles often indicate higher levels of Depression, Tension-Anxiety, Fatigue, Confusion-Bewilderment, and Total Mood Disturbance" (p. 10). In addition to assessing dimensions likely to be affected by the diagnosis of cancer, the POMS offers the advantage of a brief administration time, usually three to five minutes. Consequently, the inventory may be administered at the beginning of every therapy session to track changes in mood.

Scores on the POMS have been associated with survival times for cancer survivors. Hopwood and Maguire (1992), for example, found an association between longer survival times and both lower total mood disturbance and higher vigor scores on the POMS for participants of cancer support groups. Andersen, Kiecolt-Glaser, and Glaser (1994) found that for women with gynecologic cancers the POMS total mood disturbance and depression scales were significantly related to white blood cell counts.

Beck Depression Inventory

The Beck Depression Inventory (BDI), published by Psychological Corporation (San Antonio, Texas), is another useful assessment tool for cancer survivors (Burns, 1980; Golden, Gersh, & Robbins, 1992). This inventory is designed to assess the symptoms and severity of depression. It consists of twenty-one symptoms of depression; respondents indicate their experience of each of these symptoms on a 0-3 scale. Like the POMS, the administration of the BDI takes only a few minutes. It too can be administered frequently to assess changes in mood level.

State-Trait Anxiety Inventory

Next to depression, anxiety is the most commonly reported psychological symptom in cancer survivors. The inventory that seems to have been most widely used to assess anxiety in this population is the State-Trait Anxiety Inventory (STAI). Published by Consulting Psychologists Press (Palo Alto, California), this inventory consists of two twenty-item paper-pencil tests that measure enduring (trait) anxiety and immediate (state) anxiety. Completion of the inventory requires about fifteen minutes.

Cancer Inventory of Problem Situations (CIPS)

The CIPS was designed to help people with cancer identify their psychological and physical problems (Ganz, 1988; Schag, Heinrich, & Ganz, 1983). This self-administered inventory requires approximately eighteen minutes for completion and has excellent test-retest reliability and content validity. The inventory consists of 131 statements, divided into twenty-one categories of problems (activity, anxiety in medical situations, changes in physical appearance, cognitive difficulties, communication with medical staff, control in medical situations, dating relationships, domestic chores, eating, employment, finances, pain, physical abilities, prostheses, relationships with family and friends, self-care, side effects from treatment, significant relationships, sleeping, transportation, worry). People indicate on a five-point scale, ranging from not at all to very much, the extent to which each of the statements has applied to them within the past month. Three scores can be obtained from the inventory—Total Severity Rating, Total Number of Problems, and Average Intensity Rating—in addition to information on nature of perceived problems.

The goal of the authors of this inventory was to move away from assessing only the emotional impact of cancer and toward "a more specific behavioral description of problems created by the disease" (Schag, Heinrich, & Ganz, 1983, p. 23). This instrument seems useful for clinical and research purposes as well as for planning rehabilitation.

Measure of Adjustment to Cancer (MAC) Scale

The MAC scale was developed to assess adjustment to cancer, including both cognitive and behavioral responses people make to diagnosis of the disease (Watson et al., 1988). People indicate on a 1-4 scale the extent to which items on this inventory apply to them. Responses then yield scores in five categories: Fighting Spirit, Avoidance (Denial), Fatalistic (Stoic Acceptance), Helpless, and Anxious Preoccupation. The theoretical basis for this inventory is the finding by Watson and Ramirez (1991) that a fighting spirit and avoidance were associated with better adjustment to the diagnosis of cancer than were the other three categories of response. Fighting spirit and avoidance also have been associated with a longer survival time. This inventory has demonstrated good reliability and seems useful in providing a rapid assessment of attitudes and an indication of whether further psychotherapeutic intervention is needed.

Other Inventories of Transient Symptoms

Many other inventories are also cited in articles on the assessment of cancer survivors. The following list includes the most important of these:

> *Courtauld Emotional Control Scale (CECS)*. This questionnaire was designed to assess the extent to which people report con-

trolling anger, anxiety, and depression (Watson & Greer, 1983). This inventory was originally intended for use with women who had been diagnosed with breast cancer because of the demonstrated association between that diagnosis and suppression of anxiety and anger. However, the inventory also may be used with people who have been diagnosed with other types of cancer. Watson and Greer (1983, p. 305) concluded that this scale "is capable of discriminating those who report controlling emotional reactions."

Dealing with Illness Coping Inventory. This forty-eight-item questionnaire was designed to assess current cognitive and behavioral responses to illness (Fawzy et al., 1993).

Folkman and Lazarus Ways of Coping Checklist. This is yet another inventory to assess coping skills (Folkman & Lazarus, 1980).

Hamilton Rating Scale. This inventory is similar to the BDI and focuses primarily on the assessment of depression.

Hopelessness Scale. Assessment of suicidal ideation and other depressive symptoms are the focus of this inventory (Golden, Gersh, & Robbins, 1992).

Hospital Anxiety and Depression (HAD) Scale. This inventory was designed to measure anxiety and depression in a general medical and surgical population (Zigmond & Snaith, 1983).

Melzack-McGill Pain Questionnaire and the Wisconsin Brief Pain Inventory. These instruments are useful in assessing a cancer survivor's experience with pain and tracking changes in that symptom (Fischer & Corcoran, 1994; Golden, Gersh, & Robbins, 1992).

Moos Coping Scale. This is another inventory designed to assess and describe coping behaviors (Friedman et al., 1992).

Psychological Adjustment to Illness Scale. Developed primarily for use with cancer survivors, this inventory assesses how people are coping with serious illness (Derogatis, 1977).

Recognizing Your Type C Behavior. This twenty-item yes-no questionnaire was designed by Temoshok and Dreher (1992) to assess whether people have personality patterns that correspond with the Type C or cancer-prone personality.

Rotterdam Symptom Checklist. This checklist measures psychological and physical distress as well as overall quality of life in cancer survivors (de Hael, van Knippenberg, & Neijt, 1990).

Schedule for Affective Disorders and Schizophrenia (SADS). This inventory is designed to be completed by an examiner or therapist while conducting an intake interview. Published by Biometrics Research/Research Assessment and Training Unit-New York State Psychiatric Institute, this inventory facilitates assessment of psychopathology.

Symptom Checklist-90. This ninety-item self-administered checklist has been used to provide a quick assessment of the presence of psychological distress and mental disorders in cancer survivors (Derogatis et al., 1983).

Linear Analog Approach to Assessment

Several research studies have used a linear or visual analog to assess the feelings and behaviors of cancer survivors. Sutherland, Lockwood, and Cunningham (1989) translated the POMS into a linear analog format, consisting of six ten-centimeter lines with descriptive statements at either end. Respondents are instructed to make a vertical mark on each line to indicate the position that best describes how they have been feeling during the past week. The six scales include Not at all fatigued/Extremely fatigued, Not at all anxious/Extremely anxious, Not at all confused/Extremely confused, Not at all depressed/Extremely depressed, Not at all energetic/

Extremely energetic, and Not at all angry/Extremely angry. Scoring is accomplished by measuring in millimeters the distance from the end of each line that indicates an absence of symptoms to the place where the mark was made. Total mood disturbance can be computed by totaling the six measures.

The linear analog was found to provide a good assessment of dysphoric mood and to show a strong relationship to POMS scores. Greer and Burgess (1987) used a similar measure to provide a quick assessment of self-esteem. The visual analog scales can be modified to measure and track changes in many variables related to adjustment to cancer and provides reasonably accurate information despite its informal nature.

Assessment of Suicidal Ideation

Although suicide is not common among cancer survivors, it is more common than in the general population. Males with cancer are more likely to commit suicide than women. The greatest risk for suicide is shortly after the diagnosis has been made (Hughes, 1987). Determination of the presence of suicidal thinking is of course essential to effective treatment.

Breitbart, Levenson, and Passik (1993) identified the following "cancer suicide vulnerability factors" (p. 185): advanced illness and poor prognosis, uncontrolled pain, depression and hopelessness, delirium and disinhibition, loss of control and helplessness, preexisting psychopathology, prior suicide history, a family history of suicide, and exhaustion and fatigue. Isolation and abandonment have also been associated with suicidal ideation in cancer survivors. People who present with some of these signs may be at high risk for suicide and are particularly likely to need intensive psychotherapy.

Lifestyle and Health Attitudes Assessment

Both during and after the immediate crisis of cancer, assessment of people's lifestyles can be useful in helping them to make the most of the rest of their lives and improving their health-related behaviors. Research also has shown that indicators of good quality of life are associated with higher levels of natural killer cell activity (Andersen, Kiecolt-Glaser, & Glaser, 1994). Several instruments are available to assess lifestyle and health-related behaviors:

Life Assessment Questionnaire (LAQ). Developed by the National Wellness Institute (Stevens Point, Wisconsin), this inventory assesses current levels of wellness and identifies potential risks. It measures ten dimensions: physical fitness, physical-nutritional, physical–self-care, drugs and driving, social-environmental, emotional awareness, emotional control, intellectual, occupational, and spiritual areas (Elsenrath, Hettler, & Leafgreen, 1988).

Lifestyle Coping Inventory. This 142-item questionnaire, also published by the National Wellness Institute, assesses the following seven dimensions: coping style actions, nutritional actions, physical care actions, cognitive and emotional actions, low-risk actions, environmental actions, and social support actions.

Health and Daily Living Form. Developed by Moos, Cronkite, Billings, and Finney (1984), this inventory provides information on current health-related behaviors.

Millon Behavioral Health Inventory. This 150-item questionnaire, published by NCS Interpretive Scoring Systems, was developed to assess the attitudes of physically ill adults toward daily stressors, health and illness, and health care personnel, factors that are related to health outcomes (Millon, Green, & Meagher, 1982). The inventory also has been used to assess the possibility that psychosomatic reactions are contributing to a person's experience of an illness or disease.

Multidimensional Health Locus of Control Scale. This inventory was "developed to tap beliefs that the source of reinforcement for health-related behaviors is primarily internal, a matter of chance, or under the control of powerful others" (Wallston, Wallston, & Devellis, 1978, p. 160). It can facilitate understanding and prediction of health behaviors and can contribute to the effectiveness of programs designed to change behavior (Wallston, Wallston, Kaplan, & Maides, 1976).

Quality of Life Index. Completion of this inventory provides information on activities, daily living and self-care, health, support, and outlook. It has been used in cancer rehabilitation programs to help people adjust to the emotional and physical impact of cancer (Parker, Levinson, Mullooly, & Frymark, 1989).

Wellness Inventory. This 120-item inventory measures twelve dimensions: self-responsibility and love, breathing, sensing, eating, moving, feeling, thinking, playing and working, communicating, sex, finding meaning, and transcending (Palombi, 1992). It was designed to promote personal growth as well as new ways of solving problems.

Overview of Chapter

Standardized assessment of attitudes, behaviors, emotions, and symptoms can provide a clearer and deeper understanding of cancer survivors and can promote more effective treatment. The brief inventories, such as the POMS, the BDI, and the STAI, are especially appealing to clients because they facilitate self-expression and provide a measure of change. Therapists are encouraged to incorporate structured assessment into their work with cancer survivors as appropriate but should be sure that the use of these tools does not interfere with the establishment of a positive therapeutic relationship or detract from the cancer survivors' opportunity to discuss their concerns.

Effective Psychotherapy
for Cancer Survivors

Compelling research, discussed in Chapter One, has demonstrated a relationship between personality and coping mechanisms and both adjustment to cancer and the course of the disease. Adjustment to cancer, including the resumption of usual interpersonal, occupational, social, and sexual activities (Andersen, 1992), as well as alleviation of any severe emotional distress, can be facilitated through psychotherapy. Although clinicians need to be cautious about emphasizing the as yet uncertain impact of personal variables on the course of the disease, helping people to achieve behaviors and attitudes that are conducive to coping effectively with cancer can certainly improve their quality of life and that of their families and may in fact enhance their prognosis. According to LeShan (1989, p. x), "the same psychological approach that leads to the fullest effectiveness of the immune system is the approach that leads to the fullest and richest life—both during the time a person has cancer and afterward."

Goals of Psychotherapy for Cancer Survivors

Psychotherapy can help people who have had a diagnosis of cancer to achieve the following overall goals:

1. Become aware of their fears and feelings about the disease and its treatments and express them in positive ways

2. Alleviate depression, anxiety, and excessive arousal

3. Develop effective stress management skills

4. Have a sense of optimism and empowerment, a fighting spirit

5. Acquire a sense of control and self-efficacy

6. Achieve competence in communication and assertiveness skills and use them effectively with family, friends, health care providers, and others

7. Restore or establish positive family and other interpersonal relationships

8. Promote helpful use of support systems, including the therapist

9. Acquire information about their disease and its treatment options

10. Make sound decisions about treatment options as well as other issues

11. Reduce the aversive side effects of cancer treatment

12. Maintain self-concept in the face of the disease and its treatment

13. Deal successfully with spiritual or existential issues related to cancer

14. Maximize establishment of a healthy and rewarding lifestyle

15. If necessary, cope effectively with fears of recurrence and death

Psychotherapy for cancer survivors has been termed *adjuvant psychotherapy* (Moorey & Greer, 1989), because it is provided in addition to medical treatment and is designed to both supplement and complement that process. Adjuvant psychotherapy is useful not only to cancer survivors with diagnosable mental disorders but also to people who are coping reasonably well but could benefit from some therapy. According to Moorey and Greer (1989, p. 37), "there is complete agreement that patients with cancer should be viewed not as persons suffering from psychopathology but, essentially, as psychologically normal individuals under severe stress." The remainder of this chapter provides an overview of what information has been provided by research on the nature of effective psychotherapy for cancer survivors and on the stages in the counseling process.

Research on Effective Strategies for Psychotherapy with Cancer Survivors

Many programs and approaches to psychotherapy have been found to be effective in helping cancer survivors. The optimal form of therapy seems to be a multifaceted approach that affords cancer survivors the opportunity to express their feelings in an empathic, accepting, and supportive context and uses cognitive and behavioral strategies that promote effective coping, reduce arousal, enhance sense of control, and resolve specific problems.

Although the focus of treatment is primarily on present concerns, especially the disease, attention also should be paid to the past in order to address any unresolved losses, build on previous strengths, and deal with other family or individual issues that may have an impact on the current crisis. Consideration also should be given to the future; helping the cancer survivor establish a healthier and more rewarding lifestyle is not only important for its own sake but because it may reduce the chances of a recurrence or further spread of the disease.

Cognitive-behavioral therapy has been found particularly effective in reducing depression and improving body image in people with cancer (Hopwood & Maguire, 1992). In addition, such techniques as desensitization, relaxation, and visual imagery are useful in helping people deal with the treatment of cancer. Improvement of health-related behaviors such as diet, sleep, and exercise also can reduce stress and improve the immune system. Breitbart (1989) found that most cancer survivors are highly motivated to learn and practice cognitive-behavioral techniques because those techniques can restore a sense of control and personal efficacy and provide active participation in the treatment process.

Psychosocial interventions such as family or group therapy have also been found to reduce stress, enhance quality of life, and improve health behaviors and treatment compliance in cancer survivors (Andersen, Kiecolt-Glaser, & Glaser, 1994). These interventions will be discussed further in later chapters of this book.

Structured Psychotherapy Programs

Many structured programs have been developed to help cancer survivors. Some of these are ongoing programs offered through medical or psychological treatment centers. Others are time-limited, experiméntal programs, conducted to obtain information on the impact of psychotherapy on people with cancer. Both types of treatment services provide information that is useful in guiding the psychotherapy that is provided to cancer survivors.

Cunningham, Lockwood, and Cunningham (1991) developed a treatment program based on the hypothesis that perceived lack of control could contribute to the anxiety and depression experienced by many people with cancer. They designed a psychoeducational program that included seven weekly two-hour sessions focused on enhancing people's sense of control. The participants were taught coping skills, relaxation, mental imagery, stress reduction, cognitive restructuring, goal setting, and management of lifestyle changes. Following the intervention, a high correlation was found between improvements in perceived self-efficacy and improvements in both quality of life and mood. The researchers concluded that aversive stimuli, such as cancer and its consequences, were rendered less painful and disruptive if fears were diminished by perceived self-efficacy in coping.

A typical experimental intervention was described by Fawzy and Morton (1990). People with malignant melanoma were provided six weekly therapy sessions, each one and one-half hours in duration, an average of 112 days postsurgery. Therapy was conducted in small groups (seven to ten people) and included health education, problem-solving skills, stress management and relaxation, and support. Although changes were not evident at the end of the treatment, at six-month follow-up, people who had received the group treatment showed considerable improvement in use of active-behavioral coping skills and stress management as well as in immune functioning. The authors concluded that coping behavior could be learned or enhanced, stating, "The results indicate that a short-term psychiatric group intervention in patients with malignant melanoma with a good prognosis was associated with longer-term changes in affective state, coping, and the NK lymphoid cell system" (p. 729).

Further information on short-term structured interventions is provided by the work of Edgar, Rosberger, and Nowlis (1992). Their approach to psychotherapy with cancer survivors targeted three areas: increasing knowledge, enhancing personal control and strengthening coping, and reducing emotional arousal. Techniques used included setting graduated and attainable goals, teaching problem-solving skills, cognitive appraisal and reframing, relaxation, and visualization. Treatment was provided to people with various types of cancer over five one-hour sessions.

The above study is particularly important because of the information it yielded on the connection between the timing of treatment and its impact. Follow-up studies of people who received an early intervention (EI = average of 10.8 weeks after their diagnosis) and those who received a later intervention (LI = average of 28.2 weeks after diagnosis) indicated that both groups manifested a similar and moderate decline in depression over the first four months following the psychotherapy. However, in the next four months, the LI group showed significantly less depression and anxiety, fewer intrusive thoughts, and a greater sense of self-control. Between eight and twelve months after treatment, both groups continued to improve, but the LI group maintained an edge over the EI group. The researchers explained this finding by stating that during the first few months after diagnosis, people focus primarily on existential, life-or-death issues and may feel too overwhelmed to derive much benefit from coping-skills training. Their primary need is for basic support. However, once the initial fears have subsided, people will have an increased readiness to benefit from structured cognitive-behavioral treatment. Edgar, Rosberger, and Nowlis recommended using those interventions not immediately after the diagnosis but rather several months later. They also pointed out that the changes resulting from psychotherapy continue and may even accelerate months after psychotherapy has been completed. The authors found particularly strong support for behaviorially oriented programs involving active goal setting and stress reduction. Their review of multiple studies of the use of psychotherapy with people with cancer indicated that treatment incorporating behavioral techniques yielded better results than purely supportive interventions.

Psychotherapy seems helpful not only in reducing targeted symptoms but also in modifying personality styles and attitudes that have been associated with the incidence and prognosis of cancer. Greer et al. (1992) provided six one-hour sessions of individual cognitive-behavioral therapy to 174 people with cancer who had a life expectancy of at least one year and who manifested "psychological morbidity" (p. 676). Spouses sometimes were included in the therapy. At the end of treatment, the people in the experimental group had significantly higher scores in fighting spirit and significantly lower scores in helplessness, anxious preoccupation, and fatalism, as well as anxiety and other psychological symptoms. The percentage of people who were severely anxious declined from 46 percent to 20 percent in the experimental group and from 48 percent to 41 percent in the control group while the percentage who were depressed declined from 40 percent to 13 percent in the experimental group and from 30 percent to 29 percent in the control group. These changes persisted at a four-month follow-up.

In another review article (Trijsburg, van Knippenberg, & Rijpma, 1992), critical analysis of twenty-two studies indicated that nineteen out of twenty-two demonstrated the positive impact of providing psychological interventions to cancer survivors. That article found that individualized counseling was particularly helpful in relieving distress, improving self-esteem, and establishing a sense of control. It also alleviated physical problems (nausea, fatigue, weight loss) and improved activity level and sexual relations. Structured counseling was highly effective in reducing depression, distress, and anxiety and in improving self-concept. Behavioral interventions and hypnosis were very helpful in reducing anxiety, depression, anger, hostility, confusion, and distress, as well as pain, nausea, and vomiting related to cancer treatments.

Bos-Branolte (1987) conducted an experimental study to compare individual and group psychotherapy for cancer survivors, with both offering primarily cognitive-behavioral techniques. Nine months after the intervention, both groups, composed of women with gynecological cancers, demonstrated improvement in self-esteem, sense of well-being, body image, and partner relationships. However, body image and relationships improved more in those people who received individual therapy.

Another study (Watson, Denton, Baum, & Greer, 1988), providing counseling to women with breast cancer, sought to make help available at particularly stressful times. The counselor was present when the physician informed the woman of the diagnosis, met with her at her home prior to surgery, saw the woman at the hospital both before and after her surgery, and then made a follow-up visit to the home several weeks later. Counseling was subsequently provided as needed. Treatment was present-oriented, emphasizing crisis intervention, and including emotional support, information, and practical advice on prostheses, as well as help with adjustment. At three months postsurgery, the experimental group was significantly less depressed than the control group and had a greater sense of self-efficacy. Adjustment of people in the treatment group continued to surpass that of the control group until one year after surgery when the two groups were no longer significantly different.

Comprehensive Treatment Programs

Comprehensive and intensive treatment programs provide another avenue to helping people deal with cancer. These programs often are residential and may involve family members as well as cancer survivors. Both Lawrence LeShan in Florida and the Simontons in California, well known in the field of psychotherapy for people with cancer, have such programs. The Simontons' program is typical of these multifaceted and comprehensive programs (Simonton, Matthews-Simonton, & Creighton, 1992). It involves eleven major forms of intervention:

1. Helping people identify major stressors they experienced in the six to eighteen months prior to diagnosis
2. Exploring the possible benefits or secondary gains of the illness
3. Relaxation
4. Mental imagery
5. Overcoming resentment
6. Setting goals and planning for the future
7. Finding an inner guide
8. Managing pain
9. Exercise
10. Coping with fear of recurrence and death
11. Developing family support

The elements in this program encompass many of the ingredients that should be included in any psychotherapy for cancer survivors.

Summary of Findings

Studies of the use of psychotherapy with cancer survivors overwhelmingly support the positive impact of treatment. Although a small number of clinicians have alleged that attending to the psychological adjustment of people with cancer "produces rather than discloses symptoms, this is a specious argument for which there is absolutely no evidence" (Moorey & Greer, 1989, p. x). This information, as well as the research indicating a high incidence of psychological upset in response to cancer and the beneficial effects of even brief psychotherapy with cancer survivors, suggests that whenever possible the emotional needs of cancer survivors should be assessed and psychotherapy offered to them in addition to their medical treatments. Therapy should be presented not as another remedy for pathology but rather as a vehicle to promote health and growth as well as develop coping skills. As Temoshok and Dreher (1992, p. 82) put it, psychotherapy can help cancer survivors to embark on "a path of transformation with hope but without illusions." A comprehensive and holistic approach to treatment that emphasizes support as well as cognitive-behavioral approaches to combat stress and improve fighting spirit and sense of control seems most effective in helping cancer survivors move forward on that path. There is some indication that individual therapy seems superior to group therapy in alleviating the distressing symptoms of cancer survivors. In addition, timing of interventions is an important factor; supportive interventions are especially important in the initial stages of dealing with cancer while cognitive-behavioral interventions become more important later.

Psychotherapy for Each Stage of Cancer Survivorship

Although a cancer survivor may seek psychotherapy at any point, including initial diagnosis, treatment, recovery, or recurrence, the usual time to seek help is early in the process, during the struggle to come to terms with the diagnosis. The most common presenting concerns of survivors include fear and anxiety, depression, and concern for their children (Jevne, 1990). Other common presenting concerns include anger, pain, dissatisfaction with their medical care, tension, insomnia, guilt, hopelessness, powerlessness, resentment, marital difficulties, issues around treatment compliance, lack of motivation, and suicidal ideation. Of course, clinicians need to adapt the process of psychotherapy so that it addresses the special needs and difficulties of the particular person. At the same time, a series of predictable stages in counseling cancer survivors has been identified. These stages bear considerable similarity to Kübler-Ross's five stages of dying: denial, anger, bargaining, depression, and acceptance (Winograd, 1992). Awareness of these stages can help both clinicians and clients to have a sense of direction in therapy and to move through a process that will address the multiple and changing needs of the cancer survivor.

Stage 1: Coming to Terms with the Diagnosis

Stage 1 commonly encompasses three phases of emotional reactions: anxious uncertainty prior to the diagnosis, then shock and denial, followed by distress and depression, after the diagnosis has been made.

Prediagnosis: Anxious Uncertainty

People's initial responses to a diagnosis of cancer have much to do with whether they had symptoms that troubled them prior to the diagnosis, what their interpretation of those symptoms was, and how surprising the final diagnosis was. If there had been symptoms—a lump in the breast, a persistent cough, or changes in the color or shape of a mole, for example—the person may have suspected the presence of cancer long before the diagnosis was made. For most, it will still be a shock, a devastating piece of information. However, for others, the diagnosis may bring a sense of relief, that finally the cause of their symptoms has been identified and treatment can begin. One cancer survivor who had attributed her symptoms to

HIV was initially relieved at the diagnosis of a cancer with an optimistic prognosis.

The diagnosis is likely to be particularly difficult when it comes as a complete surprise, such as the woman who is told that suspicious calcifications have shown up on her mammogram or the man whose symptoms of prostate cancer are found in a routine examination. The period between the awareness of symptoms or suspicious medical findings and the ultimate diagnosis is likely to be fraught with extreme worry and anxiety. Some cancer survivors describe this as the most difficult stage in the whole process.

Psychotherapy that is initiated before the definitive diagnosis is made certainly would focus on this period of anxious uncertainty. Resolving their fears early in their illness seems to help people address their disease with greater strength and hopefulness (Winograd, 1992). However, people do not usually initiate cancer-related psychotherapy before the diagnosis is made. Because this prediagnosis phase is typically so difficult, it should be processed even after it is over.

Initial Diagnosis: Shock and Denial

Once the diagnosis is made, most people enter a phase of shock, numbness, and denial (Barraclough, 1994). Some people I have counseled have fainted when the diagnosis was given, spent several days crying uncontrollably, or withdrew and refused to discuss the diagnosis or their treatment options. Of course, other people are able to control their feelings and begin to address the disease immediately. However, they too commonly experience initial shock and disbelief. Extreme reactions are not limited to people with previous pathology; even well-functioning people with good resources may respond to the diagnosis in extreme ways.

Acute Distress and Depression

The initial reactions of disbelief and denial are short-lived for most people. The next phase typically is characterized by acute distress including high anxiety, anger, protest, and bargaining ("If I survive this, I'll change my eating habits and stop smoking"). Guilt and depression also are common during this stage and are likely to persist into the next phase. These upsetting feelings may be compounded by exhaustion and physical discomfort. Family members too may be fatigued and experiencing role overload.

Once again, this phase typically is short-lived and after a few weeks the anxiety diminishes while the depression and despair increase (Barraclough, 1994). The future seems bleak during this phase and thoughts of death as the inevitable outcome of the disease are common. People may withdraw, grieve for themselves and the families they think they will leave behind, and have difficulty believing even their physicians, who may emphasize that their prognosis is positive. Some people have troubling spiritual or existential concerns.

Psychotherapy During Stage 1

People who are in the early stages of coping with a diagnosis of cancer typically will benefit most from psychotherapy that provides support as well as help with decision making. Initially, people may seem to become more tense and depressed as a result of therapy as they review their experience with cancer and explore their feelings (Bloom, Ross, & Burnell, 1978). However, positive changes in mood, anxiety level, and sense of control and self-efficacy generally will be observed within several sessions.

Providing Support

Support gives cancer survivors the strength they need to address their disease effectively. It helps them see that they are not alone in their fight, that their reactions are appropriate and understandable, and that they can mobilize their resources and develop a fighting spirit. The following interventions are useful in communicating this support:

Telling their story. Most cancer survivors have a compelling need to tell the story of their disease for many months, to review the symptoms, to talk about the way the diagnosis was made, to review their reactions and those of people who are close to them, and to explore the meaning cancer has for them. Beginning the process of psychotherapy with cancer survivors by helping them tell their story will go a long way toward building rapport and helping them digest and make sense of what has happened. Journal writing between therapy sessions can be invaluable in helping people process what they are experiencing.

Empathy and acceptance. Communicating the core therapeutic conditions of understanding and positive regard are critical in the early stages of psychotherapy with cancer survivors. Their sense of self, their world, and their very lives are already threatened. The clinical setting should afford them a place where they can find comfort and security, where they can really express and show their feelings. Borysenko (1988, p. 163) captured well the accepting stance of the therapist when she wrote, "The only negative emotions are emotions that you will not allow yourself or someone else to experience." Denial, misinterpretations, strong displays of anger, and even hopelessness should *initially* be accepted with understanding, warmth, and concern. However, if these attitudes become chronic, disabling, and interfere with treatment, they should be addressed (Temoshok & Dreher, 1992). Cancer survivors' self-acceptance is also important and may be facilitated by affirmations, self-care, and acceptance by others.

Development of outside support systems. Cancer survivors as well as their close family and friends need a great deal of outside support. This can come from support systems the survivor already has in place. Therapists can have joint sessions with the cancer survivor and appropriate friends and family. Those close to the survivor may be experiencing their own anxiety and depression in response to the diagnosis and might benefit from some counseling. In addition, therapists can coach both the survivors and their important friends and family members on how to best support each other, maintain open communication, and go on with their lives.

Structured support groups, such as those offered by the American Cancer Society or cancer treatment centers, also can be very helpful. Although survivors may have difficulty being with other people who have cancer, particularly if those people are doing worse than they are, the benefits of a peer support group seem to outweigh the drawbacks for most people. The opportunity to share feelings and experiences with other cancer survivors can help to normalize reactions, to enable people to believe that finally someone really understands them, to demystify the process of diagnosing and treating cancer by hearing the experiences of others, to gather information on choices and coping skills, and to develop a bond with others who share their disease. Therapists can encourage their clients to become involved in structured support groups by reviewing their benefits and providing information on contacts and resources.

Exploration of factors that might facilitate or interfere with the person's efforts to cope effectively with cancer. In order to maximize the help therapists can offer, they should gather information about such factors as experiences with illness, ways of coping with previous crises, family functioning, and current lifestyle that will have an impact on the cancer survivors' efforts to deal with the present stressor. The importance of these factors was discussed further in Chapter Two.

Facilitating Decision Making

Regardless of their degree of emotional upset, most people who are diagnosed with cancer will soon have to gather information and make decisions about their treatment. From a therapeutic point of view, postponing these decisions until the person has moved past the initial stages of shock and acute distress might seem advisable. However, from a medical point of view, that usually is not possible. Therapeutic interventions can facilitate this process of decision making in several ways:

Information gathering. Before cancer survivors can make sound decisions, they must have accurate and adequate information about the particular nature of their disease, its prognosis, and their treatment options. The oncologist or oncological surgeon usually will be the first and primary source of that information. Therapists can help clients to develop, organize, write down, and ask questions of their physicians so that they have a clear picture of their disease. Using lists and schedules can help the cancer survivor to feel organized, grounded, and in control and can provide direction and reassurance. In most cases, therapists should gently encourage their clients to obtain information from multiple sources of information including printed material as well as physicians. Second and even third or fourth opinions from physicians can help people obtain full information and make wiser decisions. Helping clients identify sources of information, specifying their questions, and perhaps encouraging involvement of family and friends in the information gathering can facilitate that process. Therapists also may decide to communicate directly with physicians and oncologists, with their clients' permission, to clarify their own understanding of the medical situation, to join forces with the medical team, and to facilitate client-physician dialogue. This topic will be discussed further in Chapter Ten.

Empowering the cancer survivor. Through the support they receive, their growing ability to manage and accept their feelings, and involvement in the process of information gathering, most cancer survivors will find they are regaining or developing a sense of self-efficacy. They begin to hope that indeed they can marshal the inner resources and professional help they will need to defeat the disease. This feeling of empowerment is an integral ingredient in the development of a fighting spirit and can be nurtured by encouraging cancer survivors to establish small, manageable goals that are relevant to coping with cancer and then mobilize themselves to achieve those goals. While it is important not to add to the survivor's sense of being overwhelmed, dividing tasks into manageable steps and encouraging some action on the part of the survivor can promote needed self-confidence as well as mastery of necessary activities.

Making decisions. Finally, decisions regarding treatment must be made. Therapists can help cancer survivors and if appropriate their family members to make those decisions in a thoughtful, rational way. Information needs to be assessed and organized, conflicts or discrepancies need to be explored and resolved if possible, and pros and cons of each option need to be weighed. Examining alternatives in terms of both their medical consequences and the impact they are likely to have on the person's quality of life, both in the short run and over time, is particularly important. Then, if the impact of a medically sound choice seems overwhelming, therapists can help people to find compromises or develop support systems and coping mechanisms that will enable them to deal with the aversive consequences of such a medical treatment.

Stage 2: Adjustment and Acceptance

Most cancer survivors will move through the early reactions of shock and acute distress within a matter of several weeks. Increasingly, they accept the diagnosis and incorporate it into their lives, particularly if they have received some help from therapists, family, and friends. However, underlying depression and even despair is common during this period as well as bouts of increased arousal and anxiety. Cancer survivors may feel vulnerable and lonely during this stage and have a strong sense of loss. Life as they knew it may seem to have vanished and they are left confused and without clear direction or a vision of the future.

Most cancer survivors continue to need help during this stage. However, their needs are different than they were in the first stage.

Counseling the Cancer Survivor in Stage 2

Goals of counseling cancer survivors who are struggling to accept and cope with the diagnosis and treatment of cancer and to reduce their feelings of depression and perhaps anxiety include the following:

Modify dysfunctional thoughts. Recently diagnosed cancer survivors often have rigid and pessimistic beliefs about the course of their disease and the impact it will have on them. Identifying and disputing these irrational and persistent thoughts can reduce depression and anxiety and promote a sense of empowerment. Cognitive techniques can be effective in accomplishing these goals.

Promote relaxation and stress reduction. Behavioral techniques, such as progressive muscle relaxation, biofeedback, and an increased activity level, and cognitive-behavioral techniques, such as stress inoculation and systematic desensitization, can reduce the tension and anxiety that often accompany the diagnosis and treatment of cancer.

Facilitate the process of treatment. According to Barraclough (1994, p. 8), "All anticancer treatments have unwanted physical side effects." The standard treatments—surgery, chemotherapy, and radiation—can have a powerful aversive impact on the cancer survivor. Common side effects range from the short-term, uncomfortable ones (such as hair loss, nausea, and vomiting) to the permanent and disabling ones (loss of body parts, vision, or normal speaking voice). Psychotherapy at this point can facilitate adjustment to these difficult changes as well as actually ameliorate the severity of such side effects as nausea and pain. Specific techniques to accomplish these goals will be discussed later in this book.

Continue development of a fighting spirit. Maximizing the cancer survivor's sense of control and involvement in the treatment process can contribute to the maintenance or development of a fighting spirit and a sense of empowerment, important in promoting both emotional and physical health. Cancer survivors may not be able to exert much direct control over their medical condition, but they can control their reactions. Techniques such as imagery and assertiveness can contribute to the development of a fighting spirit and may improve immune system functioning.

Promote cohesiveness, support, open communication, and a return to relatively normal functioning in the family. Focusing on family members as well as on cancer survivors seems important at this stage. The high stress of stage 1 may have led cancer survivors to abandon their usual activities, to conceal fears and reactions from others, and to neglect close friends or family members. Now is the time to reverse those patterns, to restore usual family rituals and schedules as much as possible, and to attend to the needs of the healthier members of the family, while at the same time maintaining the support they are providing the survivors.

Stage 3: The Aftermath of Cancer

Cancer is both an acute and a chronic disease. Even when people have successfully passed through the acute phases of diagnosis and treatment of their disease and are beginning to think of themselves as healthy, the possibility of recurrence and the emotional and physical consequences of the disease and its treatment remain. Of course, if the treatment has not been successful, the survivors and their family may need to deal with additional treatments, deterioration, and eventual death from the disease. Both groups may need to mourn their physical and emotional losses, particularly the loss of the belief in a long and healthy future. Cancer survivors may be relieved at the end of their treatments and yet fearful now that they are on their own and do not have the sense of security that can be provided by regular treatments and contact with the medical team.

The remainder of this chapter will provide an overview of the third or chronic stage. More detailed information on this stage and psychotherapy with people in this stage is contained in Chapters Eleven and Twelve of this book.

Counseling the Cancer Survivor in Stage 3

Psychotherapy can help cancer survivors in this stage in the following ways:

Coping with the enduring side effects of the disease. Changes in fertility, sexual desire, physical and cognitive functioning all may have resulted from cancer and its treatment. Clinicians can help by encouraging people to recognize, express, and manage their feelings about these negative changes; promote positive but open family communication about role changes and altered functioning; encourage adequate medical care for the side effects; and use cognitive and behavioral techniques to maximize functioning and reduce irrational thinking about the impairment ("No one will ever marry me with one breast").

Establishing a healthy lifestyle. Relationships have been demonstrated between such behaviors as smoking, eating a high-fat diet, and excessive exposure to the sun and incidence of cancer. Developing a healthy lifestyle can reduce the likelihood of recurrence or the development of another cancer. Such a lifestyle also can contribute to a reduction in depression and promote a sense of mastery, an overall sense of self-esteem and well-being, and a sense of healing, both emotionally and physically.

Maintaining/establishing a rewarding quality of life. Regardless of how much longer cancer survivors will live, therapists can help them to identify what they want to accomplish in their remaining time and what will make the rest of their lives rewarding. Cancer often serves as a turning point, leading people to reevaluate their lives and beliefs and make personal, spiritual, and lifestyle changes that will be rewarding to them. People with a positive prognosis may make significant changes in their career and family lives as they resume the roles and activities they had before the diagnosis of cancer. Some may continue their involvement with cancer in a positive way, volunteering to help others or becoming activists to raise awareness and funding for cancer research. Even those with a short time to live sometimes make major changes in their priorities and relationships.

Helping people deal with both the fear and the reality of recurrence and death. Even for cancer survivors who are not coping with a recurrence or metastasis of cancer, fear lingers and is reactivated by minor symptoms, anniversaries, and deaths and recurrences of other survivors. Psychotherapy can help people manage these fears and address them in constructive and realistic ways. For those people actually dealing with a recurrence or metastasis, the challenges are many. Their struggles may resemble those of cancer survivors in stages 1 and 2 discussed above but are likely to be far more difficult, both physically and emotionally. Family members too are likely to need even more help in coping with the disease and if necessary the death of a loved one. Later chapters in this book will discuss these issues further.

Overview of Chapter

The most effective approach to psychotherapy for people with cancer seems to be what Lazarus called "technical eclecticism," in which cognitive-behavioral techniques predominate but are incorporated into a flexible framework that provides considerable empathy and support and is adapted to the needs of the individual (Golden, Gersh, & Robbins, 1992). Treatment should be holistic and comprehensive, including family and friends as indicated and emphasizing health and positive coping rather than illness. For most people, treatment will be relatively brief, perhaps six to thirty sessions (Haber, 1993), but duration of treatment too needs to be tailored to the needs of the individual. The remaining chapters in this book focus primarily on techniques and other important information that will guide therapists working with cancer survivors. Chapters Five and Six will provide information on cognitive, behavioral, and expressive interventions, essential ingredients in the treatment of cancer survivors.

5

Cognitive Psychotherapy

Approaches to psychotherapy that have been shown to be helpful to cancer survivors include cognitive, behavioral, and affective interventions. This chapter will focus on cognitive interventions, including stress inoculation, modifying dysfunctional thinking, decision making and problem solving, imagery, meditation and mindfulness, hypnotherapy, affirmations, use of dreams, journal writing, and bibliotherapy.

Rationale for Providing Cognitive Therapy

Cognitive therapy is especially appropriate for cancer survivors. Misconceptions and fears associated with the diagnosis of cancer may contribute to the development of extreme thoughts of hopelessness, suffering, and death. These thoughts can make coping with an already difficult situation even more difficult. As Moorey and Greer (1989, p. 57) stated, "How he or she thinks about the illness and its implications for his or her life is central to adjustment."

Witmer, Rich, Barcikowski, and Mague (1983) identified the following five beliefs as being strongly associated with the combination of high anxiety and physical illness:

1. The past continues to influence me so much that it is hard for me to change or prevent bad things from happening.

2. I can't help getting down on myself when I fail at something or when something goes wrong.

3. It is very important for me to be liked and loved by almost everyone I meet.

4. I must be perfectly competent, adequate, and achieving in all that I do to consider myself worthwhile.

5. I have little control over my moods, which are caused mostly by events outside myself.

For cancer survivors, negative thinking is most common in the following five areas (Mathieson & Stam, 1991):

1. Fear of recurrence

2. Feeling different or damaged

3. Expecting to be rejected by others

4. Communicating with health care providers

5. Concern about lifestyle changes

Cognitive therapy addresses dysfunctional thoughts in a fast-paced and structured fashion that is likely to promote optimism and empowerment in the cancer survivor as well as involvement in the treatment process.

Moorey and Greer's Model

Moorey and Greer (1989) developed a model for providing adjuvant psychotherapy to cancer survivors based on a combination of Beck's cognitive therapy (Beck, Rush, Shaw, & Emery, 1979) and behavioral psychotherapy. Their treatment approach was designed for anyone having difficulty coping with a diagnosis of cancer and sought to promote a positive fighting spirit and a sense of personal control, to reduce emotional distress, to develop effective coping strategies, to allow self-expression, to improve communication between the survivor and others, to promote treatment compliance, and to reduce the side effects of treatment. Moorey and Greer's clients received six to twelve one-hour sessions of structured therapy that was problem oriented, teaching people how thoughts contribute to distress and how they could reduce their distress by modifying their thoughts. Tasks were suggested for completion between sessions to accelerate the therapeutic process.

Although Moorey and Greer emphasized the importance of therapists developing rapport and collaboration with the cancer survivor and allowing some time for ventilation of feelings, the first few sessions focused on teaching the cognitive model as well as identifying strengths and problems. Relevant readings and other tasks between sessions were recommended from the outset.

The middle phase of therapy involved monitoring thoughts, reality testing, replacing inaccurate and dysfunctional thoughts with ones that were more accurate and constructive, and problem solving. Sessions were carefully planned and typically began with a review of the homework that was completed between sessions. Behavioral techniques were integrated into the model to increase activity level and sense of mastery.

The final phase of treatment focused on relapse prevention. Therapy in that phase emphasized building coping skills, addressing fears of recurrence and death, exploring underlying assumptions about the future, and facilitating any necessary future planning and lifestyle changes.

Identifying and Modifying Cognitive Distortions

Many cancer survivors have negative and automatic cognitions about the reasons for their disease, its prognosis, its treatments, and their own reactions and behaviors. These thoughts can be elicited by exploring people's initial reactions to the diagnosis of cancer and their explanations of the meaning or cause of the disease.

Burns (1980) provided the following list of ten major types of cognitive distortions. This list and accompanying examples, expressed by cancer survivors, may be useful for teaching survivors about cognitive distortion.

1. *All-or-nothing thinking*: "I have cancer. I'm going to die."

2. *Overgeneralization*: "The doctors had a hard time doing a biopsy on the lump in my breast and then it was malignant. I just know the surgery will be painful, I'll throw up all through chemotherapy and then it won't work. I'll be dead before I'm fifty."

3. *Mental filter*: "The doctors said I have a good prognosis but I had those two positive lymph nodes. The cancer probably has spread throughout my body and they just haven't found it yet."

4. *Disqualifying the positive*: "Yes, I know most of the people in my support group are doing very well but this one woman had a cancer like mine and now she has metastases to her brain and her liver. I'm sure I'll wind up like that too."

5. *Jumping to conclusions*: "My oncologist didn't return my telephone call yesterday. She probably has bad news and doesn't want to tell me."

6. *Magnification*: "I keep remembering that I fainted when they told me I had cancer. I thought I was a strong person but I guess I'm not. I'm so ashamed that the doctor and my wife saw me pass out."

7. *Emotional reasoning*: "My mother died a terrible death from cancer and I'm a lot like her. The doctors say things look good but they can't really know. I'm sure I'll wind up like her."

8. *"Should" statements*: "I should be strong for my husband. I can't let him or the children know how I really feel. They're already so upset."

9. *Labeling and mislabeling:* "I'm a loser. Nothing has ever gone my way and this won't either."

10. *Personalization:* "I knew I shouldn't have eaten all that fast food. That must be why I have cancer."

Once the cognitive distortions have been identified, they can be written down and addressed. Burns suggested the following six steps, illustrated by examples relevant to cancer survivors:

1. Describe the situation that led up to an unpleasant feeling: Husband tells wife that she should stop crying and feeling sorry for herself, that she'll never get well unless she develops a fighting spirit.

2. Identify and rate degree of emotion on a percentage scale of 1-100 percent: discouraged, 95 percent; angry at myself, 60 percent.

3. Write the automatic thoughts: "I can't do anything right. First I get cancer and now I'm so pessimistic, I'll never get that fighting spirit that I need to survive."

4. Identify the nature of the distortions: all-or-nothing thinking, personalization, disqualifying the positive.

5. Develop and write a rational response: "Of course, I feel sad and upset that I have cancer, but that doesn't mean I'm not fighting. I'll be getting chemotherapy, I've been reading books about cancer, and I'm seeing a therapist to help me cope with the disease."

6. Identify and rate resulting emotions: discouraged, 50 percent; angry at myself, 10 percent; angry at my husband, 10 percent; hopeful, 25 percent.

Additional cognitive and behavioral steps can then be identified by both client and therapist to reduce the negative thinking and provide a sense of control. In the above example, the woman might plan to have a conversation with her husband about her reactions to his comment, role playing that conversation in the therapy session first so that she is clear about what she wants to say and uses communication skills that avoid blaming and open up dialogue. She also might read about exactly what it means to have a fighting spirit and can keep a diary of times when she acts, feels, or thinks in a way that reflects that spirit in order to assess whether there is any truth to her husband's statement.

The following techniques also can promote cognitive restructuring (Moorey & Greer, 1989):

Reality testing: Establish a hypothesis and assess its accuracy using past experiences, sources of information, and logic. ("I believe my prognosis is not good. I will get a second opinion, review my medical records, and do some reading to determine whether my physician is right in being optimistic.")

Seeking alternative explanations: Brainstorming other possible and more positive explanations or outcomes. ("I'm worried that my stomach pain is a sign the cancer has spread. However, my stomach might just be upset from all this worry or I might have hurt myself when I was exercising yesterday. I'll check with my doctor to see what it is.")

Decatastrophizing: Identifying a person's worst fear and then assessing its likelihood, probable impact, and possible solutions. ("My worst fear is that I will die a horrible painful death like my grandfather and leave my family in poverty. However, I know that the odds are on my side, that now very powerful medications are available to control cancer pain, and that I have life insurance and social security payments that will help my family.")

Reattribution: Recognizing that factors outside of themselves may be the cause of people's difficulties, thereby reducing feelings of self-blame. ("I feel like my bad health habits are to blame for my getting cancer, but I know that cancer is usually due to genetics and carcinogens. I guess I really didn't make myself get cancer.")

Distraction: Focusing on other thoughts and activities to prevent ruminating about cancer. (A woman with a lavish wardrobe in which she took considerable pride was encouraged to make a mental inventory of all her clothes whenever she found herself absorbed with negative thoughts of cancer.) Thought stopping, instructing oneself again and again either out loud or subvocally to stop thinking a certain thought, is a related strategy that can stop rumination.

Effective use of cognitive therapy can promote development of what Moorey and Greer (1989) called a "survival schema," an optimistic view of oneself and one's illness. Just as negative cognitions can be generalized, so can this schema so that it colors all areas of the person's life with a positive perspective.

Martin Seligman's Learned Optimism

Another perspective on cognitive therapy has been provided by Martin Seligman (1990), who developed the concept of "learned optimism." Seligman found that people have explanatory styles that influence the sense they make of events in their lives. People he described as optimists saw negative events as temporary, circumscribed, and not their fault, although they could take responsibility for positive events. They were usually unfazed by defeats but rather viewed them as challenges. Pessimists, on the other hand, manifested what Seligman termed "learned helplessness." They blamed themselves for disappointments, gave up easily, and were prone to guilt, anxiety, depression, and hopelessness. They viewed negative events as enduring and uncontrollable and positive ones as temporary. Optimists are more likely to respond to cancer with a fighting spirit whereas pessimists are prone to have a hopeless/helpless response to cancer. Particularly at risk for developing emotional disorders are people who would be classified as pessimists and who tend to ruminate, spending a great deal of time thinking about the causes and circumstances of their difficulties rather than taking effective action. (One caution emerging from Seligman's work is the finding that pessimists typically are more realistic and accurate in their appraisal of events than are optimists. Therapists should be careful lest optimists make unwise decisions that contradict medical advice.)

Seligman found that cognitive-behavioral therapy can teach pessimists to become optimists. He summarized his model in an ABCDE pattern: *adversity* leads to *beliefs* that have affective and behavioral *consequences*. Distorted beliefs should be *disputed* in order to *energize* the person.

That pessimists can become optimists is important information for cancer survivors because optimism seems to have medical as well as psychological benefits. Application of Seligman's theories to cancer survivors led him to conclude that "when tumor load is small . . . optimism might spell the difference between life and death" (p. 176). His research on the impact of twelve sessions of weekly cognitive group therapy plus relaxation on people who were diagnosed as having colon cancer or melanoma demonstrated that cognitive-behavioral therapy enhances immune activity.

Meichenbaum's Stress Inoculation Training

Another approach to cognitive therapy for cancer survivors is Meichenbaum's Stress Inoculation Training (SIT) (Meichenbaum, 1985). Meichenbaum described stress as "a cognitively mediated relational concept," reflecting the interaction between person and environment (1985, p. 3). Stress has been defined as "the perception of individuals that their life circumstances have exceeded their capacity to cope, a subjective experience" (Locke & Colligan, 1987,

p. 71). Meichenbaum suggested an approach to reducing stress that first assessed the person's appraisal of stressful events, the person's resources and options, and the nature of the stressor.

Following that assessment, appropriate coping skills were taught. Meichenbaum viewed coping as "behavioral and cognitive efforts to master, reduce, or tolerate the internal and/or external demands that are created by stressful transactions" (p. 3). People who cope through avoidance or blame are more likely to experience high stress and anxiety than are people who use active cognitive and behavioral approaches to coping (Friedman et al., 1992).

Because distorted thinking is especially likely at times of high stress, Meichenbaum's approach uses many of the approaches to modifying cognitions discussed earlier in this chapter. However, his model is particularly useful in helping people learn problem solving and decision making. SIT, like most cognitive-behavioral models, has an educational component, teaching people about the nature of stress, the transactional relationship between stress and coping, and the role that cognitions and emotions play in engendering and maintaining stress. The client's stressful thoughts and experiences are then translated into specific difficulties that are amenable to solution. For example, Theresa's general fear of her upcoming mastectomy encompassed many specific fears: that she would feel scared and helpless when she was wheeled into the operating room; that things said while she was anesthetized would have a negative impact on her; that she would be in pain after the surgery; that she would have difficulty looking at herself after the surgery; and that her partner's feelings toward her would be affected by the surgery.

Once the specific fears have been delineated, they can be rated on a scale of 1-100 subjective units of distress (SUDS). Therapy generally would begin with one of the mildest fears and aim to reduce it to a manageable level. Information could be gathered and ways to address the stressors could be developed that not only would reduce the specific fears but could be generalized to address other fears and stressors as well. This process of dividing stressful events into smaller pieces is an important tool for cancer survivors, who commonly become overwhelmed by the emotional, practical, and physical demands of their situation. Taking one day at a time or one piece at a time can make challenging situations manageable and bolster self-esteem.

An overview of the problem-solving component of SIT involves seven steps: (1) problem identification, (2) goal selection, (3) generation of alternatives, (4) evaluation of each possible solution and its probable consequences, (5) decision making and rehearsal of strategies, (6) implementation, and (6) evaluation and reinforcement of accomplishments (Meichenbaum, 1985). The combination of tools to promote both stress reduction and problem solving make SIT a powerful therapeutic approach for helping cancer survivors.

Visualization and Imagery

Visualization or imagery is another very important tool for helping people cope with cancer. Imagery can reduce anxiety and facilitate relaxation, it can promote a sense of empowerment and control, it can improve decision making and reduce confusion, it can ameliorate pain and other symptoms, it can ease discomfort associated with treatment, and perhaps it can even reduce one's chances of a metastases or recurrence of the cancer.

Encouraging Cooperation with Visualization

Although most people with cancer are eager to try any techniques that seem likely to help them, some view guided imagery and other nontraditional techniques as silly or worthless or even threatening. To encourage cooperation, people should be given a rationale for whatever process is being used and should be encouraged to approach it with a playful, curious, open attitude. Therapists might say something like, "I don't know whether guided imagery will be helpful to you but many cancer survivors find it reassuring and relaxing. I'd be curious to see how you react. How about if we try it? You can let me know if you want to stop at any point, but you may discover some new and interesting things about yourself." In addition, people should be given as much control over the process as possible and should be helped to see that this not some mysterious process that is being done to them but rather their inner resources coming to the fore. Timing of the guided imagery and its duration and intensity should be carefully adapted to the needs of the individual. Imagery is especially likely to be well received if it appeals to a person's dominant sense faculty (visual, auditory, tactile, or olfactory) (Siegel, 1990).

Visualization, relaxation, and other strategies discussed in this chapter will be most powerful if they are practiced and used between therapy sessions. Tape recordings can be made of the guided imagery sessions to be played daily as well as before stressful events to help the survivor cope more effectively. Practicing as little as three to five minutes a day, in the same, comfortable place, seems to greatly facilitate the process of visualization (Fanning, 1988). The best times to use this tool are upon awakening and before falling asleep. Keeping an arm slightly raised during the visualization can keep the person awake if that is a concern.

The Process of Guided Imagery

My own work as well as the literature suggest the following steps for using guided imagery with cancer survivors:

1. Promote relaxation using techniques discussed in Chapter Six.
2. Person imagines a peaceful, relaxing scene where he or she feels secure, whole, and healthy.
3. Wise, inner guide is accessed; means are provided in the image for the guide to appear (a path, from behind a rock, through a door). Guide offers a channel for messages from the unconscious (Fanning, 1988). The first time a possible guide appears, the person should imagine greeting the visitor and

asking whether he or she is the guide. If the answer is not affirmative, the person should ask for the guide to be sent.

4. Question or task is presented to the inner guide.

5. Guide assists person with task or question, usually either making a decision or trying to mobilize the immune system by visualizing the body destroying any remaining cancer cells.

6. Person visualizes self as healthy and successful at dealing with the task or question.

7. Guide departs. Person says goodbye, makes a statement of appreciation to the guide, and affirms that the guide can be summoned whenever it would be helpful.

8. Person gradually leaves the peaceful scene and returns to the room.

Example of Guided Imagery to Fight Cancer

The following sample illustrates a therapist taking a person through a second session of guided imagery. The nature of the guide and the imagery for the cancer cells and the immune system were based on images that arose for the client during the first imagery session.

> Now I would like you to relax your body and sink deeply into your chair. Uncross your arms and legs and gently let your eyelids close. Pay attention to your breathing and breathe deeply and from your diaphragm, in and out, in and out, feeling your diaphragm move deeply with each breath . . . take full, deep, slow breaths . . . and with each breath, you will feel all the tension, all the stress flowing away, feeling all your muscles relax, your head, your face, your shoulders, your arms, your hands, feeling the tension being released. . . . Now relax your chest, your lower body, your legs, and your feet. Feel the breath flowing through your body, relaxing all your muscles. Now when you feel ready and relaxed, I'd like you to

return to that special place, that beautiful lush forest
where you feel as strong as the strongest tree. Look
around you and you will remember how happy you feel
here, how calm and peaceful, surrounded by the tall,
green trees and the tall mountains, how happy you are
to be back here. Now as you look around, you will see
your inner guide, the fox, coming out from behind the
tree. He has been waiting for you to call on him, always
ready to help you. I'd like you to greet your guide and
when the two of you are ready, you will once again go on
a journey inside your body.

Now you are inside your body with your inner guide.
You look around and see that everything seems to be
glistening with health and strength and you believe that
you can conquer this disease. If there are any cancer cells
left, they are weak and confused, like dead leaves that
have fallen on the ground. Just to make sure you have
gotten rid of all those cancer cells, you and the fox will
marshal your immune system, the natural killer cells that
are like the woodsmen, as powerful as Paul Bunyan.
They are wearing their red jackets, the extra power they
have gotten from your chemotherapy, that red liquid that
will make your natural killer cells even stronger than
they already are. With the fox as their guide, the woodsmen will go on a search to find and destroy any of those
weak, confused cancer cells that might be left. If they
find any, they will destroy them and flush them out of
your body so that you will be healthy and free of disease.

When you and the fox are satisfied that any cancer
cells have been eradicated, I'd like you to thank your
powerful immune system, the woodsmen, for their help,
and return to the peaceful forest. It's time to say goodbye
to your guide for now but you know that he is always
there to help you and as you and he agreed, every time

you open the front door to your house, you will think of your guide and know that he is always with you.

Now look around the forest and be aware of how healthy and strong you feel, knowing that soon your treatments will be over, and you and your family can do those things you've been wanting to do, go camping, celebrate many birthdays together, and watch your daughter graduate from college. When you are ready, I'd like you to gradually come back to this room, slowly open your eyes, and remember where you are now. Now I'd like you to draw a picture of the images you had and then we can talk about what came up for you during this visualization.

This guided imagery has been carefully planned to include the following elements that seem to be important in imagery for cancer survivors:

- Relaxation

- Images that promote a sense of control, optimism, and a fighting spirit

- Reassurance, strength, and support provided by the inner guide

- Reminder of the guide's availability

- Image of the body as strong and powerful

- Image of the cancer cells as weak, small, and powerless

- Image of the immune system as able to destroy the cancer cells and flush them out of the body

- Image of treatment enhancing the body's already strong abilities to fight cancer

- Image of the person as happy and healthy, resuming a rewarding life

- Processing and reinforcing the guided imagery without judging the person, the images, or the person's success in creating images

Other Uses for Visualization

In addition to the above example, other ways of using imagery also can be helpful to the cancer survivor.

The threat and discomfort presented by an aversive treatment or medical test can be reduced by imagining the medical procedure in a way that is comical or absurd, desensitizing the person to the threat, or changing the threat into something positive. One man who found the vivid color of his chemotherapy disturbing imagined it as Kool-Aid, his favorite childhood drink, being put into his veins to make him as healthy and carefree as he had been as a child. A woman who felt claustrophobic when the equipment used in bone scans and radiotherapy was moved close to her body imagined the equipment as a large, colorful beach umbrella, protecting her from the sun. Pain that seemed to be consuming a person was imagined as getting smaller and smaller until it was the size of a raisin.

Imagery can provide a mental rehearsal for coping with challenging experiences. Meichenbaum (1985) suggested that such imagery include the experience of stress as well as successful coping with the stressor; imagining mastery or success without the presence of the stressor and the challenge of coping seems to provide a less realistic image that is not as useful. Cancer survivors can imagine a movie of themselves performing feared acts, thereby identifying and reinforcing desired behaviors. Rating their distress in terms of SUDS can indicate whether anxiety is being controlled (Golden, Gersh, & Robbins, 1992). A teenaged boy used this strategy to practice telling his friends without crying that he had cancer, something that was very important to him.

Brigham (1994) used what she called a "transformational fantasy" with cancer survivors: the therapist guides the client on a symbolic journey, typically walking down a strange road, seeing a house, and exploring the house. Dialogue used during the session encourages the person to describe and explore reactions to the scene. Brigham believed that the scene symbolized the person's life and that the house and its rooms, doors, hallways, and other features gave information about the person. This technique might be especially useful with people who are denying or suppressing their reactions to cancer; it can give people a better sense of their resources. Drawing, cutting relevant pictures from magazines, or imagining oneself as nonhuman (for example, an animal, a rosebush) are other ways to use imagery to access feelings.

Imagery can provide positive distraction. Creation of an absorbing and readily accessed fantasy or series of images can reduce rumination and provide a tool to reduce anxious images and messages.

Reliving a scene through the imagination can help people retrieve their feelings and reassess their behavior. For example, the experience of receiving the diagnosis of cancer often is so upsetting that people block out information or blame themselves for losing their self-control. Processing such an event in the mind can help people understand it more clearly and view their reactions from a different perspective ("Yes, we know that you became very distraught when you were told you had cancer but did you run out of the room screaming? Did you throw a paperweight at the doctor? No? Could it be, then, that you reacted in a very understandable way?")

Imagery, using the inner guide, can be used to find answers to difficult questions. Fanning (1988) called this "receptive visualization." The guide might be asked for advice or a dialogue with the guide can help the person explore the answers to various questions: Is a bone marrow transplant the right treatment for me now? How can I deal more effectively with chemotherapy? Should I tell my eighty-seven-year-old father that I have cancer?

McWilliams and McWilliams (1991) suggested having a person imagine hosting a "gratitude party," in which all people and events for which the person can be grateful are reviewed. This technique can promote optimism and a positive outlook as can an image that projects a person into a positive time in the future.

Research on Using Visualization with Cancer Survivors

Brigham (1994) found a strong connection between imagery and course of the disease. In her study, 93 percent of those people who were able to develop a positive image of their immune system defeating cancer recovered from the disease while 100 percent of those who could not develop such an image failed to recover. Whether this correlation reflects the power of the imagery or people's awareness of the nature of their disease has not been determined, but regardless of the reason for the correlation, imagery is an important tool in helping therapists understand and treat cancer survivors.

Using Meditation

Meditation, a procedure closely related to and often combined with visualization, is another tool that is very useful to cancer survivors. Meditation can promote a sense of physical and emotional calm and balance, can focus attention and promote insight, and can help the cancer survivor to let go of worries and fears (Smith, 1986). Meditation also can promote mindfulness, a calming attitude in which the person maintains a focus on the present and takes each day at a time, as well as feelings of being centered and self-confident (Zimpfer, 1992). It can help the cancer survivor find what Jevne (1988) called a "stillpoint," the point at which the person experiences a feeling of calm, effortlessness, and strength in the midst of a threat.

Borysenko (1988) wrote of the capacity for meditation to free the inner physician, promoting an inner state of awareness of the body's needs and facilitating healing. She stated, "The final goal of meditation is to be constantly conscious of experience so that relaxation and peace of mind become the norm rather than the exception" (p. 47).

Meditation typically is preceded by five to ten minutes of preparation that might include muscle relaxation, stretching, deep breathing, and scanning the body for particularly comfortable or uncomfortable sensations. Meditation usually is done when a person is seated in a chair in a place that is relaxing and free of distractions. Then, as Smith (1986, p. 67) wrote, "The instructions for meditation can be put very simply: Calmly attend to a simple stimulus. After every distraction, calmly return your attention—again and again and again."

According to Borysenko (1988, p. 36), "Meditation is any activity that keeps the attention pleasantly anchored in the present moment." The focus of attention might include a relaxing sound or word (such as peace or health); a visual image such as a candle, a glass of water, or a still pond; the process of breathing deeply and slowly; a mantra (a word with spiritual meaning); or a repetitive movement such as walking or swaying. The stimulus may be internal or external, passive or active, meaningful or neutral, and can involve any sense. Selection of a stimulus that is compatible with the survivor's usual style is likely to encourage involvement in meditation. For example, people who have an inner locus of control seem most receptive to an image while those with an external locus of control usually are most comfortable focusing on an object or picture.

Various types of meditations have been described:

Meditative imagery: Focusing on a relaxing mental image or picture

Transcendent imagery: Using images that encourage letting be, such as a child or the night sky

Contemplative meditation: Seeking meaning or answers by focusing on a question, memory, experience, or inner guide

Open focus meditation: Imagining oneself in a setting conducive to new ideas and experiences, then adopting a mental set of openness and receptivity and waiting to see what comes into awareness

Meditation is most helpful when it is used on a regular basis, once or twice a day for ten to twenty minutes, and it can also be used in briefer forms to promote relaxation in stressful situations. It seems to be most effective when the person is not tired; Borysenko (1988) recommended meditating before a meal. With practice, meditation usually becomes easier, deeper, and more rewarding.

People sometimes feel anxious when meditating or express concerns about their ability to meditate because they find other thoughts intruding on their concentration. They can be reassured that that is a common experience and does not detract from the value of the meditation. They also might be encouraged not to judge themselves. They just need to redirect their attention back to the stimulus whenever they realize they are distracted. However, they also should be aware of and discuss any fears that intrude on the meditation.

Other objections to meditation are that it has a religious association and that it seems like a waste of time. These objections may be countered by allowing the cancer survivor full control over the choice of a stimulus and a schedule for meditation and encouraging a "try it and let's see how it works" attitude.

Zimpfer (1992) suggested comeditation as a way of reducing resistance. In that process, the therapist breathes audibly along with the client, with the breaths serving as the focus of the meditation. This approach can promote trust, support, and rapport as well as cooperation.

However, if a person objects strongly to meditation or to any other element of adjuvant psychotherapy, that element can simply be eliminated. A rich array of tools is available to help clinicians working with cancer survivors and elimination of one or two of them is not likely to interfere with treatment.

Using Hypnosis

Hypnosis, described as "essentially a state of heightened and focused concentration" that can modify perceptions and increase suggestibility, is another useful tool for cancer survivors (Breitbart & Passik, 1993, p. 67). Used either in psychotherapy sessions or in the form of self-hypnosis, this process can have a calming effect and can increase a sense of well-being. It also can promote insight and feelings of mastery.

Several studies have illustrated the use of hypnosis with cancer survivors. Rossi (1993) found that hypnosis, using such techniques as reframing and conversion of a symptom into a signal, could improve the functioning of the immune system. Hypnosis also is useful in pain control, especially with children (Kumar, 1987), and in modifying the aversive impact of some cancer treatments. Spiegel and Bloom (1983) compared the impact of supportive group therapy with or without self-hypnosis for women with metastatic breast cancer and found that the women who received instruction in self-hypnosis not only had greater control over their pain but also reported less anxiety, depression, and fatigue than the control group. Approximately two-thirds of cancer survivors are hypnotizable and can derive some benefit from hypnosis (Breitbart, 1989). Children between the ages of five and eleven are at the peak of hypnotizability (Spiegel, 1985).

Although a review of the principles and procedures of hypnosis are beyond the scope of this book, therapists who already have training in that area or are interested in obtaining such training will have yet another tool that will be very helpful to their clients

(Jevne, 1990). Readings that are especially helpful to the therapist who wants to use hypnosis with cancer survivors include Rossi (1993) and Spiegel and Spiegel (1978).

Using Affirmations and Reframing

A group of interventions that might be called "positive self-talk" all entail, as Chandler, Holden, and Kolander (1992, p. 173) put it, "reprogramming the subconscious" to promote self-confidence and reduce the threat posed by cancer and its treatment. These interventions include affirmations, coping self-statements, reframing, and thought substitution.

Affirmations and coping self-statements are messages that cancer survivors tell themselves to promote feelings of self-efficacy. The survivors do not need to believe these messages initially; they only need to be willing to repeat them frequently to themselves. Posting the messages where they will see them, such as on the refrigerator, in the car, or on the bathroom mirror, can further strengthen the impact of the message. Messages might be general ("I am strong and confident") or specific, perhaps transforming a problem into a challenge ("I will breeze through this surgery and return home as soon as I can"). Through practicing these affirmations, first within the therapy session and later outside of the sessions, people often come to believe the messages and are better able to cope with cancer.

Reframing and thought substitution involve replacing a negative, discouraging thought with one that is optimistic and empowering. For example, instead of thinking, "How I dread Tuesdays, my chemotherapy day," someone might be encouraged to think, "This Tuesday means one less chemotherapy treatment. I can't wait for these Tuesdays to pass. I know I can handle it—I only have four more."

All forms of coping self-statements seem most effective if the messages are generated by the cancer survivors and are put in personally meaningful terms. The messages should be repeated many times each day, especially to interrupt and deflect fears and pessimistic ruminations (Meichenbaum, 1985). In that way, negative automatic thoughts can be replaced by positive ones.

Using Dreams

Accessing dreams, experienced either while awake (daydreams) or while asleep, can provide another source of information and help. Siegel (1990) found that dreams of cancer survivors often provided clues to their physical and emotional health. As Schlossberg (1984, p. 25) stated, "The dreams—our imagined possibilities of what may be—are a key to our identity."

Dreams can be explored to reduce denial and increase awareness of feelings. A Gestalt approach to a discussion of dreams, in which the client assumes the roles of various parts of the dreams and describes what each feature looks like, feels like, and wants to say, is a particularly useful and nonthreatening approach to understanding dreams. In this way, the meaning of the parts of the dream will come directly from the client rather than from the therapist. In addition, dreams that are not positive can be redone in a waking state to reduce the depressing impact of the dream, create hope of a different outcome, and identify resources that might prevent the dream from coming true (Borysenko, 1988).

Using Reading and Writing

Many cancer survivors find it helpful to keep a journal of their feelings and reactions to the diagnosis and treatment of their disease. This may be done as a planned and structured activity, on an as-needed basis, or in the form of automatic writing (Spencer & Adams, 1990), in which the person writes rapidly and spontaneously, allowing any feelings or thoughts to be expressed without regard to grammar, sentence structure, or other constraints. The journal also might take the form of a stress diary, in which the person lists stressors, their circumstances, their level of severity, and the person's thoughts, feelings, and behaviors in response (Golden, Gersh, & Robbins, 1992). Writing a weekly progress report of one's efforts to deal with cancer and regain health can be empowering and can give a sense of accomplishment. McWilliams and McWilliams (1991) suggested emphasizing accomplishments and positive experiences by writing them down and posting them; negative thoughts and reactions might be written down and burned, while the person imagines the pessimistic thoughts or disappointing experiences disappearing in the flames.

The process of writing not only helps cancer survivors to become more aware of their feelings and more able to express those feelings but also helps to reduce fear and anxiety. Somehow, the process of writing about troubling or frightening experiences seems to encapsulate and externalize them and allows the cancer survivor to have a greater sense of control over and distance from upsetting emotions. Pennebaker (1990) believed that honest disclosure of thoughts and feelings in a journal could also improve mood, health, and immune functioning.

List making is another process that can be helpful. Cancer survivors often feel inundated by all the decisions they need to make and all the tasks they need to complete, including medical visits, treatments, filing claims for medical insurance, dealing with the bills, and helping family members handle the illness, in addition to their usual responsibilities. Making lists that prioritize tasks and schedule them in a realistic way can reduce the pressure on cancer survivors and can help them to believe that indeed they can do everything that must be done even though some of the nonessential activities may be neglected. Scheduling also gives the message that the great stress associated with the initial diagnosis and treatment of cancer is time limited and resumption of life as it was before cancer might be possible. Lists can also be used to record troubling thoughts and plan time to think about them later; this can reduce negative ruminating and help the person put the thoughts in proper perspective (Seligman, 1990b).

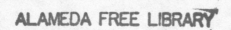

Bibliotherapy is another helpful approach. Reading books with information about cancer and its treatment, particularly accounts of people who have dealt with cancer successfully, can be encouraging. The combination of education and psychotherapy seems especially powerful in reducing distress and promoting healing (Ganz, 1988). Also beneficial is reading that helps cancer survivors develop skills that will give them a greater sense of self-efficacy and complement the process of psychotherapy; such readings might, for example, focus on communication skills, assertiveness, family dynamics, and the role of diet and exercise in good health.

Readings, as well as other activities chosen by cancer survivors, should be selected carefully so that they empower rather than depress. One woman, hoping to have a diverting night out with her husband following her recent biopsy and diagnosis of cancer, inadvertently went to see a film that dealt with a man who had been widowed by his wife's death from cancer.

Similarly, many cancer-related books that appear to be encouraging often have a negative impact on cancer survivors. Books that focus primarily on stories of miraculous recoveries of people with cancer who had the right attitude can be discouraging and can add one more source of pressure to cancer survivors who may believe that they must have such an attitude to survive. Consequently, book recommendations should be made with care and readings should be discussed in therapy sessions, with particular effort being paid to address any negative impact of ostensibly encouraging books.

Overview of Chapter

Clearly, a wealth of cognitive techniques are available that are likely to be helpful to cancer survivors. Techniques discussed in this chapter can dispel misconceptions and fears people have about cancer and can promote effective coping. The active and fast-paced nature of most of these techniques promotes optimism as well as feelings of control and empowerment in cancer survivors as they become participants in their treatment. Cognitive therapy can help people develop a fighting spirit and may even enhance prognosis. Cognitive techniques such as guided imagery and meditation, discussed in this chapter, often are combined with behavioral and affective approaches reviewed in the next chapter.

6

· ·

Behavioral and Other Approaches to Psychotherapy

This chapter reviews relevant behavioral interventions, including relaxation, systematic desensitization, development of assertiveness and communication skills, planned use of activities, exercise and diet, laughter and play. Some attention will also be given to affective approaches, including existential psychotherapy, art and other expressive therapies, spirituality, and therapeutic touch.

Behavior Therapy

Along with cognitive therapy, behavior therapy is an essential ingredient of psychotherapy for cancer survivors. The two approaches are often combined into a package that is very effective in alleviating depression and anxiety and helping survivors assess their situations clearly but optimistically and take appropriate action. Cancer survivors seem especially receptive to behavioral interventions because they can be continued between sessions, thereby providing a sense of control over the disease, a feeling of accomplishment, and a distraction from unproductive worrying.

Stress

Selye (1976) studied people's reactions to prolonged and severe stress and identified a three-stage reaction process he called the

General Adaptation Syndrome. When stress is initially experienced, people react with alarm and arousal. The second stage of reactions to stress, resistance, is the body's effort to combat the stressor. Finally, if the stressor does not abate soon and the arousal becomes chronic, the body moves into a stage of exhaustion.

Research (discussed in Chapter One) has found a positive correlation between the experience of prolonged, uncontrolled stress and both the incidence and severity of cancer. Of course, cancer itself is a significant stressor over which people have only limited control. The fear sparked by a diagnosis of cancer can immobilize the body with stress (Winograd, 1992). In addition, more than 50 percent of people undergoing treatment for cancer develop phobic-like behavioral problems including anticipatory nausea and vomiting associated with chemotherapy, anxiety associated with medical procedures, and difficulty with sleep (Redd, 1988). Consequently, those people for whom stress is likely to be harmful are exposed to highly aversive stressors through the diagnosis and treatment of cancer. Stress reduction, then, that seeks to maintain a physiologically steady state regardless of external changes is an important element of psychotherapy with cancer survivors (Rossi, 1993).

Behavior therapy is a powerful approach to stress management. Grossarth-Maticek and Eysenck (1989) studied the impact of thirty hours of behavior therapy (relaxation training plus desensitization) on women with metastatic breast cancer and found that behavior therapy was more effective in prolonging life than was no treatment, chemotherapy alone, or psychodynamic therapy. The combination of behavior therapy and chemotherapy was particularly powerful. They concluded, "Behavior therapy, by altering an individual's reaction to stress and increasing his ability to cope with the stress, significantly alters the capacity of the immune system to kill cancer cells, as indicated by the increased percentage of lymphocytes" (p. 320).

A wide variety of effective behavioral techniques are appropriate for use with cancer survivors including relaxation, systematic desensitization and stress inoculation, training in assertiveness and communication skills, modeling, behavioral rehearsal, biofeedback, activities and behavioral distraction, as well as exercise and dietary changes. Cooperation with these interventions can be maximized by presenting them as a new skill that may take time to learn, explaining why the skill is a useful one for cancer survivors, demonstrating that tension and relaxation are incompatible, fostering realistic expectations and a nonjudgmental attitude, forewarning people of the sensations they are likely to experience, and giving them permission to stop the activity before it is completed if they become uncomfortable. Behavioral interventions seem to be particularly well accepted by people who are action oriented and who may not have much facility in identifying and expressing their feelings.

Promoting Relaxation

One of the primary goals of therapy with cancer survivors is promoting what Benson (1979) called the "relaxation response." This is a profound state of rest that can be elicited by any form of mental concentration that distracts people from their cares and concerns. Borysenko (1988) described this as a neutral gear, as opposed to the usual fight-or-flight response to stress that is like passing gear. In the fight-or-flight state, stress hormones are released to provide quick energy and facilitate a rapid response. However, two of these hormones, adrenaline and cortisol, inhibit the immune system. This state therefore can be very harmful to the person who is fighting cancer, particularly if the stressor is prolonged and is accompanied by feelings of helplessness and passivity. Several behavioral approaches have been found effective in inducing a relaxation response.

Abdominal Breathing

Breathing deeply, so that the diaphragm expands with each breath, supplies the body with more oxygen and can promote relaxation. Concentration to enhance relaxation and slow breathing can be encouraged by suggesting the person count up to eight with each breath (Golden, Gersh, & Robbins, 1992). Exhaling fully through the mouth can be effective in initiating abdominal breathing. Then, shifting over to breathing through the nose can maintain the relaxing breathing. Practicing this exercise twice a day for several minutes can promote relaxation. LeShan (1989) believed that frequent use of the simple process of becoming aware of one's breathing could promote a sense of control and mindfulness as well as physical and emotional health.

Progressive Muscle Relaxation

This is a systematic approach to tensing and relaxing the muscles in sequence. Progressive muscle relaxation (PMR) can be combined with abdominal breathing; the muscles are tensed with the inhaled breath, the tension is maintained for a few seconds while holding one's breath, and then is relaxed on the exhale. Typically, PMR begins by stretching and relaxing the feet, then the legs, the buttocks, the hands and arms, the chest and shoulders, the neck, and the facial muscles. As each part is tensed and relaxed, directions focus attention on sensations of warmth, heaviness, and relaxation (Haber, 1993).

Related techniques, using breathing and PMR to promote relaxation, include sighing and yawning, head rolls, and shoulder shrugs. The body scan, suggested by Ornish (Moyers, 1993), is a more passive approach to muscle relaxation: the person lies down and, while focusing on breathing, mentally scans the body beginning with the toes. This process of becoming aware of body sensations can take thirty to forty-five minutes and seems to relax as well as focus the mind. Another approach to passive relaxation has been called "letting go" (Golden, Gersh, & Robbins, 1992). Muscles are relaxed sequentially without first being tensed.

Centering

Another technique, described as follows by Haber (1993, p. 93), is centering:

Stand with your feet about 10 inches apart, knees bent in what skiers call the "snowplow" position. Keeping your knees bent, allow your body to fall forward until your head is hanging down as close as possible to your feet. Breathe deeply. Using your fingertips to maintain your balance, and keeping your knees bent, slowly raise your heels off the ground. Experience the vibrations that go through your legs and into your body as you do this. Stay this way for as long as you can, and then slowly return your heels to the ground, keeping your knees bent. Slowly raise your upper body to an upright position and then raise your arms above your head. Explore the space around you and become aware of the space you own in the world. As you do this, stay in touch with your own inner center, and say out loud if possible, "I'm alive!"

Combining Relaxation and Imagery

Instructions for relaxation, like those for meditation, can be tape recorded for use at home to promote frequent use of these strategies. Instructions that combine relaxation with imagery are particularly powerful in promoting deep relaxation and concentration (Horowitz & Breitbart, 1993). The combination can reduce sleeping and eating problems and has been found to be as effective as medication in reducing mild to moderate anxiety. Use of PMR, diaphragmatic breathing, and visualization of a peaceful scene fifteen minutes a day for six weeks has been shown to effect significant improvement in mood (Bridge, Benson, Pietroni, & Priest, 1988).

Facilitating Acclimation to Stress

Stressors cannot be avoided. This is particularly true for people coping with the diagnosis and treatment of cancer. Although strategies such as cognitive restructuring can help moderate an overreaction to an event, behavioral techniques may be more useful in addressing reactions to undeniable stressors.

Stress Inoculation Training

Meichenbaum (1985) developed an approach he called Stress Inoculation Training (SIT). SIT combines cognitive and behavioral techniques in a program that is designed to protect people from the harsh impact that stressors can have. Using graded exposure, or gradually increasing involvement with stressors, people's fears are slowly reduced and their coping mechanisms strengthened. Information on the cognitive component of SIT was presented in the previous chapter.

Meichenbaum identified three phases to SIT:

1. *Conceptualization:* The approach is explained, client's cooperation is enlisted, and the problem is explored.

2. *Skills acquisition and rehearsal:* Depending on the nature of the stressors, the second phase would emphasize instrumental/problem-focused coping or palliative/emotion-focused techniques. The instrumental approach might include such techniques as information gathering, problem solving, communication skills training, time management, and lifestyle changes. The palliative approach would include techniques such as searching for meaning, distraction, ventilation, and relaxation. Imagery, behavioral rehearsal, coping self-talk, and graduated practice are important elements in both approaches.

3. *Application and follow-through:* The last phase of SIT is particularly important in helping people anticipate and plan to deal with setbacks and generalize the strategies to other stressful areas of their lives.

The following steps are typical of the overall process of SIT:

1. Acquaint person with strategies of SIT.

2. Assess demands of present situation and current coping skills.

3. Set concrete realistic goals, dividing stressors into manageable tasks.

4. Gather information on the stressor and how others have coped with it.

5. Generate a wide range of alternative courses of action.

6. Evaluate possibilities, determine most viable strategies, and rehearse or practice them.

7. Reward self for trying and for any success.

8. View any disappointments as a source of feedback and return to the list of alternative courses of action.

The following example illustrates the use of SIT with Marcy, a woman who recently learned that her breast cancer had metastasized to several sites in her body, including her bones. She was very apprehensive about the pain she had heard was associated with bone cancer and was overwhelmed by conflicting information she had received on treatment options. One cancer treatment center encouraged her to have a bone marrow transplant that posed some risk of death as well as some hope of a cure while another treatment center encouraged her to take a less aggressive approach that would slow down the progression of the disease but was unlikely to lead to a cure.

First, the strategies and logic of SIT were presented to Marcy, especially decision making, guided imagery, and relaxation.

Then, how much time Marcy could safely delay her decision was determined and coping skills she had used during other stressful situations, including her initial diagnosis of cancer, the death of a sibling, and a miscarriage, were explored and reinforced.

After that, goals were determined, including making a decision about treatment, reducing fears of pain, and controlling anxiety during medical visits.

Marcy developed and followed through on a plan to obtain more information. She consulted two other cancer treatment centers and spoke with people who had experienced both types of treatment that had been suggested to her. She gathered information on the impact of bone cancer and on ways to control its pain. In therapy, she was taught relaxation and imagery; a tape was made of her relaxation and imagery training so she could practice those skills at home.

Based on the information she had gathered, Marcy listed as clearly as possible her treatment options. She also developed a list of ways to combat anxiety and her fear of pain.

Decision-making skills, along with affective techniques, were used to help Marcy arrive at the decision that she would pursue the most aggressive treatment available to her. She also formulated strategies for communicating her decision to her family, all of whom were not in agreement with her choice. She practiced talking with her family and continued her use of relaxation and imagery, focusing those strategies specifically on dealing with her anticipated treatment.

Marcy developed affirmations to encourage and reward herself. In addition, she planned some pleasurable activities with her husband and with friends; those activities also served as rewards and helped to distract Marcy from her anxieties.

Finally, Marcy evaluated the success of her efforts, paying particular attention to times when her anxiety management strategies had not been effective, in order to further improve her coping skills.

Systematic Desensitization

SIT is similar to a technique called "systematic desensitization," often used in the treatment of phobias as well as with cancer survivors. Systematic desensitization can be accomplished through the use of the imagination (imaginal) or through actual exposure to the feared context (*in vivo*). For example, a combination of imaginal and *in vivo* desensitization may be used with someone who is apprehensive about beginning chemotherapy. The process would begin by teaching the person an effective relaxation strategy such as progressive muscle relaxation. Then an anxiety hierarchy would be developed, a list of fear-provoking stimuli, rank ordered according to the amount of fear each provokes. Next, exposure to the stimuli would be introduced, beginning with the least fearful and moving through the list, always pairing exposure to the feared stimulus with relaxation.

In the above example, exposure first would be imaginal. The person might imagine, in a gradual, step-by-step fashion, the experience of a successful chemotherapy treatment: visualizing the room, the nurses, the process of sitting in a special chair, extending the arm, the needle prick that will allow the infusion of the cancer-fighting fluids, the administration of the cancer-fighting drugs, the removal of the needle, and finally the act of arising, feeling healthy and optimistic. A second phase of the treatment might take place in the context of the medical facility where the chemotherapy will take place and would use *in vivo* desensitization. Again, proceeding gradually, step by step, therapist and client visit the facility, become oriented to the waiting room, meet the treatment team, explore the room where the chemotherapy will be given, and finally observe someone receiving chemotherapy. Videotapes of the client or another receiving chemotherapy can also be included in the treatment as a way to desensitize fears as well as rehearse and reinforce positive behaviors.

This process must be carefully planned so that it does not raise anxiety but rather promotes feelings of self-confidence, optimism, and control. Continuing the desensitization between sessions, with the help of a friend or family member who has been coached by the therapist, can contribute further to those positive feelings and can help those close to the cancer survivor to have a sense of contributing to the person's treatment.

Distraction

Behavioral changes that distract and shift focus also can reduce fears. For example, Helen dreaded her frequent blood tests, always done by the same grim and often rough technician. She and the therapist developed a plan in which Helen would try to make the technician smile by counteracting the technician's stony silence with warmth and praise. This focused Helen's attention off of the uncomfortable procedure she feared and onto a more positive activity. In addition, after a few blood tests, the technician began to recognize Helen and to respond to her friendliness, making the procedure a less formidable one.

Normalizing Fears

Cancer survivors often criticize themselves for being fearful of their treatments, believing they should strive to be stoic and show no fear. Normalizing their fears and helping them recognize that true bravery is facing one's fears and moving forward despite the fears can counteract this self-blame. With young cancer survivors (or adults with a sense of humor), their bravery in accepting feared treatments may be tangibly rewarded with gold stars or stickers that they can proudly display to others.

Improving Communication Skills

Having effective communication skills can enable cancer survivors to receive the help and treatment they need. Effective communication with medical staff can maximize survivors' ability to ask and receive answers to their questions, obtain understanding of their treatment options and of the likely difficulties and side effects of their treatments, and ensure that those concerns are properly addressed. Clear and open communication with family and friends can promote a sense of support and a sharing of needs and feelings.

Assertive communication may be an area of weakness for some cancer survivors: "Researchers have found that cancer-prone individuals are less assertive, suppress negative emotions, and are more willing to accept outside authority" (Golden, Gersh, & Robbins, 1992, p. 22). Even for people with satisfactory assertiveness skills, the need to express oneself clearly, set limits, and ask for help from health care professionals and concerned friends and family members can be challenging. In addition, the feelings of anger that understandably often accompany the grief associated with cancer can interfere with efforts at congruent and clear communication.

Several models are available for teaching effective communication. Books on assertiveness training such as *Your Perfect Right* (Alberti & Emmons, 1990) and *The Assertive Woman* (Phelps & Austin, 1987) provide help in identifying one's rights and wants and communicating them in a clear and nonthreatening fashion. Books on general communication such as *Straight Talk* (Miller, Wackman, Nunnally, & Saline, 1982) are also useful. Texts such as these provide examples and exercises to facilitate practice between sessions. In addition to readings and direct instructions, therapists can promote effective communication skills through modeling and demonstrations, role playing with clients, and helping them identify other people they might use as role models. Acting as if they are an assertive person they know and admire often confers the skill and confidence of that person to the cancer survivor, at least for a short time.

The following are important principles of communication to stress with cancer survivors, as well as examples of how each principle might be reflected in the words of a cancer survivor:

> *Clarification of questions, wants, and feelings:* "I want to find out why I have had this pain in my side for so long and whether it might indicate a spread of the cancer."

> *Congruence of affect, behavior, and words:* "I will let the doctor know that I am concerned and upset and need her help. I will not play down my concern to avoid bothering the doctor."

> *Keeping focus on the self, using "I" statements:* "I am very worried about the meaning of this pain and I want to know its cause" is likely to be better received than "You brush me off whenever I ask about the pain in my side. You're not much help to me."

> *Controlling emotions so that they do not detract from communication:* "Although I feel scared by the pain, I will try not to break down in the doctor's office. If I do, I will either ask for a few

minutes to collect myself or arrange to see the doctor again later."

Listening carefully to the other person: "I will take notes on the information I am given, restate that information to the doctor to be sure I understand it, and ask questions if anything doesn't make sense to me."

Demonstrating empathy or understanding of the other person: "I will let the doctor know I realize she is very busy and has limited time to spend with me. Because of that, I will be clear and direct but will not waver in making my needs known."

Willingness to negotiate or compromise: "If the doctor is too busy to spend much time with me today, I will ask for a time later this week when she can give me a full examination and listen to a description of my symptoms."

Use of consequences if no progress is being made: "If the doctor does not help me solve this problem soon, I will let her know that I will change doctors unless she does and I will do so if I don't see the doctor taking me seriously."

Planning difficult communications using role play, rehearsal with a tape recorder and a mirror to observe body language, and scripts or lists of important points: "I will make a list of my symptoms and questions and bring the list with me to the doctor."

Skill in communication and assertiveness certainly is important in helping cancer survivors cope effectively and confidently with the immediate demands of their illness. In addition, these skills are likely to have long-range benefits in their relationships, their ability to take control of their lives, and perhaps in their health.

Biofeedback

Biofeedback also can be useful in therapy with cancer survivors. Instruments are used to monitor certain bodily functions and provide feedback on those functions via a tone or light. Biofeedback can enable people to change many physical states once viewed as involuntary such as heart rate, pulse rate, muscle tension, skin temperature, and sweat-gland activity (Simonton, Matthews-Simonton, & Creighton, 1992). Breitbart (1989) found that both temperature and electromyographic (EMG) biofeedback are effective with cancer survivors in teaching relaxation and promoting pain control.

In an experimental study, Davis (1986) assigned women who had recently been diagnosed with early-stage breast cancer to one of three groups. Group 1 received EMG and thermal biofeedback while being taught progressive muscle relaxation. Group 2 received cognitive therapy, focusing on improving the participants' ability to cope with stress. Group 3 received no treatment. Immediately following the eight-week intervention, more than 25 percent of those in groups 1 and 2 demonstrated a significant reduction in anxiety while none of those people in group 3 showed anxiety reduction. These findings persisted at an eight-month follow-up.

Activities and Exercise

Cancer survivors who maximize their activity levels, particularly if they are involved in physical exercise, can derive several benefits from that process. Research has shown that physical exercise can reduce depression, increase the secretion of endorphins that can improve sense of well-being and reduce pain, and enhance the immune system by increasing the production of interleukin and the growth rate of T and B cells (Locke & Colligan, 1987; Winograd, 1992). In addition, physical activity can distract people (positive avoidance) and prevent ruminating; it can increase feelings of self-efficacy, motivation, and accomplishment; it can remind survivors that their lives can still be full and rewarding despite cancer; and it can enhance the immune system and improve overall health. Heim (1991) found that overall adjustment following a diagnosis of cancer was related to involvement in diverting activities. In addition, frequency of involving, expressive activities both at home (entertaining, hobbies, games) and away from home (meetings, seeing friends, entertainment) was correlated with likelihood of disease-free survival in women who had been diagnosed with breast cancer (Hislop, Waxler, Coldman, Elmwood, & Kan, 1987).

Certain strategies can promote cancer survivors' positive use of activities (Moorey & Greer, 1989). Cancer survivors, with the help of their therapists, can develop a list of activities they think they might enjoy and be able to accomplish in light of their medical condition. Frivolous pastimes, as well as those that are constructive, should be encouraged. Not only are they distracting, but Norman Cousins (1989) powerfully demonstrated the impact such activities can have on health. Cousins believed that watching humorous films like those of the Marx Brothers helped him overcome a painful illness.

Some cancer survivors are reassured by taking steps to plan for a recurrence of their disease. They may want to make a living or traditional will, set up a trust fund for their children, or even plan their funeral. Such activities need not be depressing or discouraging if an attitude of "hope for the best but prepare for the worst" can be maintained.

Establishing positive health habits should receive attention when activities are planned. When confronted with the many demands of dealing with cancer, people sometimes neglect their self-care or believe that they are going to die anyway so do not maintain previous positive behaviors. Eating well may be particularly difficult because of the impact of treatment on appetite. However, such habits as eliminating smoking; reducing fat, alcohol, and caffeine in the diet; increasing consumption of whole grains, fruits, and vegetables (especially cruciferous vegetables such as cabbage, broccoli, brussels sprouts, and cauliflower); and getting adequate amounts of vitamins that have been associated with a reduced risk of cancer seem particularly important.

Once a list of activities has been developed, each activity then can be rated on a 1-10 scale for the amount of pleasure and sense of mastery or accomplishment it is likely to provide. Those activities with high ratings in both pleasure and mastery are especially likely to be helpful (Burns, 1980) as are activities that increase sense of control by providing a positive distraction and building on a person's strengths. Scheduling activities increases the likelihood that they will be performed and can be especially helpful to people who feel pessimistic and helpless. If they visualize themselves succeeding and enjoying activities, this can also improve the probability that they will perform those activities.

Activities can also be used as a reward or reinforcement. Planning favorite activities for difficult times such as during the fatigue that often sets in a week or so after a chemotherapy treatment can reduce the negative impact of that difficult time. George, who was having difficulty with weight loss and nausea, rewarded himself with a meal at his favorite restaurant four or five days after each chemotherapy treatment when his appetite began to return.

For people who are resistant to increasing their activity levels, therapists might present graded task assignments, beginning with simple, time-limited, and rewarding activities (take a walk to the variety store two blocks away and buy a magazine that interests you) and gradually increasing the demands of the task to achieve realistic goals. Tasks should only be encouraged if they are clearly within the clients' abilities and are agreeable to them. Cancer survivors already have many disappointments and challenges in their lives and should not be given tasks that may lead to failure or disappointment. To ensure that outside activities and tasks are not harmful, they should be discussed and processed in the sessions. Keeping a list of accomplishments can help people to see that they are making progress and taking steps to help themselves.

"Change the Image or the Action"

Clearly, a broad range of cognitive and behavioral interventions are available that are likely to be of benefit to cancer survivors. They can all be summed up by the statement, "Change the image or the action" (McWilliams & McWilliams, 1991, p. 451). Either strategy can have a profound impact on mood, outlook, coping skills, and health.

Expressive and Other Approaches

Although cognitive and behavioral models seem most useful in therapy with cancer survivors, strategies drawn from existential, humanistic, and person-centered approaches to therapy also can be helpful and can complement the cognitive and behavioral strategies. Expressive interventions are likely to be especially welcome to people who are aware of their feelings and can express them easily. At the same time, if the interventions are chosen carefully, they may be even more beneficial to people who tend to deny, avoid, or suppress their emotions.

Expressive Therapies

Expressive approaches to therapy, interventions using art, music, and other creative forms of self-expression, have an important place in treatment of cancer survivors for several reasons:

- These approaches provide another vehicle for promoting awareness of feelings and solidifying gains and insights.

- They may reduce resistance to conventional therapy, particularly for people who find talking about cancer to be painful and difficult.

- Expressive therapies can enliven and energize the psychotherapy process.

- Expressive therapies mesh well with some cognitive-behavioral techniques such as visualization and meditation.

Although specialized training in art or music therapy certainly would be helpful to therapists, such training does not seem essential to use expressive therapies with cancer survivors because the goal generally is not to release and process deeply repressed unconscious material but rather to facilitate expression of feelings that are close to the surface. Therapists who are not well trained in these modalities should of course be aware of their own limitations.

The following are examples of ways to use expressive therapies with cancer survivors:

• Drawing a picture of their cancer being attacked by their immune system can serve both as a vehicle for exploring feelings and beliefs about cancer and a way of reinforcing a positive outlook. This technique can be used in conjunction with imagery, with the drawing reflecting the images of the inner guide, the cancer cells, and the cells of the immune system.

• Unstructured drawing, in which people are asked to simply draw what they are feeling, can relieve an impasse or give a sense of control over emotions that might otherwise seem unmanageable. Mask making or assembling collages from pictures clipped from magazines are other artistic ways to express and manage emotions.

• Pictures illustrating people coping with the challenges posed by cancer have been used successfully as a stimulus for discussion, self-exploration, and problem solving (Fawzy et al., 1990).

• Music can be used in the background during relaxation or meditation and can establish a mood that will facilitate letting go and immersing oneself in the experience. That same music can be used between sessions as a cue to help people relax or meditate on their own. Other sources of sound, such as drumming, also can be helpful and empowering.

• People might be asked to bring in music that is meaningful to them and that expresses their feelings. Playing and discussing that music in sessions can be fruitful.

• Cancer survivors who have found certain pieces of music to be reassuring and relaxing have brought tapes of those pieces with them to surgical or medical procedures and have asked that those tapes be played during the procedure. This can be especially useful in reducing discomfort for people going through magnetic resonance imagery in which they are exposed to loud noises while enclosed in a small space.

• Writing, also discussed in Chapter Five, can serve as another way to promote self-expression. The writing may take the form of a structured, daily journal of experiences and reactions or may involve freewriting, in which the person rapidly writes down words, phrases, or sentences as they arise in response to specific questions or topics such as "what I fear" or "what I want to do before I die."

Rico (1991) suggested many creative approaches to freewriting: a word sketch, two to ten minutes of writing designed to name and organize emotions; word sculptures, doodling pictures and words to create an image and release feelings; clustering, beginning with a seed word or phrase such as *I am* or *if* or *stuck/flow* and then branching off to other words that are triggered, with the new words themselves being the triggers for other words or concepts; and making lists (such as guilt lists, blame lists, happy lists).

Several of my clients, both former teachers, responded well to assignments of essays they would write on particular topics such as "How Cancer Has Affected My Life" and "How I Can Help Myself Cope with Cancer." Composing letters that may or may not be mailed uses writing to deal with unfinished business and if possible to promote communication.

• Poems and short pieces of writing by others that are meaningful can also promote self-awareness and self-expression. The poems or essays may be brought in by the clients or by the therapist. Many first-person narratives are available that describe people's efforts to deal with cancer. These can be inspiring and encouraging. However, they should be selected with care and processed in therapy sessions.

• Laughter and play, both as part of therapy sessions and away from sessions, can be both emotionally and physically healing. Laughter promotes muscular relaxation, increases pain thresholds, reduces depression and anxiety, and seems to increase natural killer cell activity (Brigham, 1994). It also can help people to access their natural, curious, and powerful inner child, a potential source of strength. Films and readings can promote feelings of pleasure as can telling jokes and other rewarding activities. All of these can serve as positive distractions from illness. Asking "What has brought you pleasure in the past?" or "What have you always wanted to do but never did?" can yield useful information on activities likely to be joyful and rewarding. Often, cancer survivors and their families become so caught up in the tasks of dealing with cancer that they neglect their usual activities and enjoyments. Encouragement from a therapist, even an assignment to have a family outing or a date, can relieve guilt feelings the people might have had at spending time in what might seem like frivolous ways.

Psychodrama or other approaches to enactment of experiences also can be fruitful, particularly in group or family counseling settings. Participants can assume roles and act out either past events, such as receiving the diagnosis of cancer, or anticipated events, such as receiving chemotherapy.

The body is another vehicle for self-expression via such experiences as massage, yoga, therapeutic touch, running, dance, or other structured or unstructured approaches to body work.

Empathy

The importance of demonstrating empathy for and understanding of cancer survivors cannot be overemphasized. Empathy, communicated primarily through therapists' reflections of people's feelings and other person-centered techniques, helps the survivors see that they have assistance and support in their fight against cancer and that others can grasp what they are going through.

Empathy is also important in promoting the survivors' awareness of their own experiences. Temoshok and Dreher (1992) found it was common for cancer survivors to have difficulty identifying and differentiating their emotions. The expressive activities discussed above will be especially useful and meaningful if they are processed in the therapy sessions and used as vehicles for labeling and exploring feelings. Recognizing and addressing anger is important because cancer survivors often suppress or avoid expressions of anger. Guilt, shame, and resentment are other emotions that often plague cancer survivors. Once strong feelings have been identified, they can be expressed, redirected, or controlled via planned self-expression, but that cannot happen until the emotions are acknowledged.

Existential Psychotherapy

Understandably, cancer survivors often reflect on the meaning and value of their lives and may feel that the door to the future has been closed for them. Callan (1989) wrote about the importance of maintaining hope in people, even when prospects for a long future are discouraging. Using the framework of Viktor Frankl's (1963) system of logotherapy, Callan helped cancer survivors discover their own reasons for living in the face of life-threatening illness and concluded, "Human beings have an amazing capacity to sustain optimism even when their expectations are regularly disappointed" (p. 36). Meaning in people's lives can be discovered by using a life review or assessment to explore such areas as religious faith, goals and aspirations, philosophy of life, interpersonal relationships, and sources of pride. Affirming a sense of meaning in one's life can promote hope as well as a feeling of mastery or personal control.

Hope is most empowering when it is based on reality. Although for cancer survivors, hope will probably include hope for a cure, it also might include hope for more immediate and attainable goals such as closer family relationships, and might also be manifested in transcendent hope based on a person's belief system. Development of goals or hopes beyond recovery from disease can be encouraged by asking, "In addition to hoping for a cure, what other things can you hope for now?"

Callan found an existential approach to be especially suitable for people who are insight oriented, but insight is not needed to benefit from activities such as guided reminiscences, writing a letter to a loved one (perhaps to be left for a child to read years later), organizing a photo album, or making a video or audio tape. All these accomplishments give a sense of meaning to life.

Spirituality

Although a structured, existential approach may not be appropriate for use with all cancer survivors, nearly all can benefit from some discussion of their spiritual feelings and beliefs. Zimpfer (1992) wrote about the tendency for cancer survivors to blame themselves for their disease and to lose faith. He encouraged cancer survivors to develop prayers that are consistent with their belief systems. These seem most powerful if they focus on self-empowerment rather than a specific outcome such as a cure. Siegel (1990) advanced the idea of forming a healing partnership with God, and Temoshok and Dreher (1992) emphasized the importance of having an active faith in which people feel a sense of power and control rather than a passive faith that involves a fatalistic belief system.

Addressing spiritual areas through guided imagery can be especially powerful. Brigham (1994), for example, suggested a guided imagery that leads people through the process of dying and death, reviewing their feelings about their lives and concluding with an opportunity to return and make changes. These types of activities can also promote discussion of very difficult topics such as one's own death or that of a loved one and what that will be like and how it will be handled, both in emotional and practical terms.

Of course, therapists focusing on people's spiritual beliefs and values should be careful not to make judgments or to give the message that people should have faith or should increase their involvement with formal religion. Intrinsic religion has been found to be significantly more strongly associated with hope and a sense of spiritual well-being than has extrinsic religion (Mickley, Soeken, & Belcher, 1992). A strong belief in something, be it formal religion, the self, the family, the medical treatment, or the harmony of the universe, seems important in helping people cope effectively with cancer (Borysenko, 1988).

Psychodynamic Psychotherapy

Although therapy for cancer survivors generally will have an active, structured, and present-oriented framework, brief psychodynamic psychotherapy also seems to have a possible role in the treatment process, either alone or integrated with other approaches. Barraclough (1994) suggested that such processes as working through guilt and loss, linking past and present issues, interpretation, identifying and modifying defense mechanisms, exploring dreams, addressing resistance, and examining transference and countertransference all have a place in therapy with cancer survivors. Attention to the inner child also may be useful; Brigham (1994) suggested helping people formulate affirmations that say what they wish they had heard from their parents. Unlike conventional psychodynamic therapy, goals would not emphasize personality change but rather would focus on empowerment and support (Haber, 1993). Psychodynamic psychotherapy can also encourage a sense of inner peace by enabling people to let go of past resentments and obligations (Zimpfer, 1992).

Medication

Some clinicians raise the possibility of using medication to ameliorate severe anxiety and depression in cancer survivors who are not responding to psychotherapy. Psychotropic medication seems to be underutilized with cancer survivors for several reasons: their depression may be disregarded because it is such a common and understandable response to cancer, the survivors may be reluctant to express suicidal and other strong feelings, adding one more drug to the treatment regimen of someone undergoing chemotherapy may seem undesirable, and oncology staff may be unfamiliar with appropriate medications (Hopwood & Maguire, 1992). However, psychotherapists who are not physicians might consider making a referral to a psychiatrist to assess the appropriateness of using medication to alleviate severe psychological symptoms.

Overview of Chapter

A broad and diverse array of treatment modalities and interventions show promise for helping cancer survivors. Therapists should be careful not to inundate their clients with too many different approaches. Instead, they should conduct a careful assessment of their clients' needs and strengths and work closely with their clients to determine those approaches that are most likely to address those needs and to be compatible with the clients' personality and lifestyle.

7

Helping People Cope with Cancer

Chapters Five and Six provided general information about the theoretical approaches and interventions that have been shown to be beneficial to people who are coping with cancer. This chapter focuses on using psychotherapy to ameliorate the impact of cancer and its treatment, including initial diagnosis, hospitalization and surgery, chemotherapy, radiotherapy, other invasive tests and treatments, short-term physical changes, long-term physical changes, changes in sexuality, and pain. Interventions that have been effective in addressing each of these aspects of cancer will be reviewed. These interventions can make an important difference: "For cancer patients, quality of life is highly dependent on the alleviation of distressing physical and psychological symptoms" (Breitbart & Holland, 1993, p. xvii).

Diagnosis

Initial reactions to a diagnosis of cancer are quite varied and may include avoidance and denial, hopelessness and helplessness, anxious preoccupation, fatalism, and, what seems to be the most positive response, a fighting spirit (Barraclough, 1994). Common emotions include bewilderment and confusion, fatigue and inertia, anxiety, anger, depression, and guilt. Many cancer survivors experience what has been called "existential plight" (Andersen, 1992) in which their whole view of life and its meaning is thrown into a state of turmoil. Anxiety is higher at the time of the initial diagnosis than at any other time in the treatment of cancer, except if the cancer recurs (Kumar, 1987). Although the nature of a particular person's reaction to the diagnosis is difficult to predict, what can be predicted with some certainty is that cancer will have a profound impact on the person's life.

Crisis Intervention

The Chinese character for "crisis" combines the characters for danger and opportunity and a diagnosis of cancer certainly offers both. A crisis intervention approach, at the outset of treatment, can help people handle the danger effectively. Adams (1991) described a typical approach to crisis intervention as including the following twelve steps:

1. Identifying who is in crisis

2. Assessing the symptoms of the crisis reaction

3. Determining the precipitant for the crisis

4. Exploring the meaning the precipitant has for the person in crisis

5. Understanding how the current crisis is linked to past experiences

6. Identifying past coping mechanisms

7. Figuring out what is preventing those coping mechanisms from being used successfully now

8. Understanding how past and present issues have combined to lead to the present emotional response

9. Promoting understanding of the situation, its implications and significance for the person

10. Facilitating exploration and integration of emotional responses to the precipitant

11. Developing and mobilizing coping resources

12. Consolidating gains, to promote effective coping with future crises

Adjusting to Personal Transitions

Spencer and Adams (1990) identified seven stages of adjustment to personal transitions:

1. Losing focus, numbness, unreality

2. Minimizing the impact, denial, even euphoria

3. Hitting bottom: depression, powerlessness, anger, sadness, self-doubting, questioning

4. Letting go of the past, forgiveness of self and others, some optimism

5. Testing the limits: energy, enthusiasm, self-confidence

6. Searching for meaning: trying to make sense of the change, relating it to one's life as a whole, introspection, reflection

7. Integrating: gaining more confidence, other areas of life resume importance

While few people with cancer will experience all these stages in sequential order, the stages provide a framework for describing how a person is coping with cancer and for normalizing those reactions.

Cancer survivors seen for psychotherapy soon after the diagnosis typically need help with the following:

Identifying, expressing, and understanding their reactions to the diagnosis. The words of cancer survivors capture best some reactions to the diagnosis of their disease:

"I never knew I could cry as hard as I did; sounds came from me that surprised me."

"Suddenly the fragility of life became starkly apparent."

"My self-esteem and self-image dropped to zero. I felt like a leper."

"I found the diagnosis and treatment of cancer to be dehumanizing."

"I remember screaming at my oncologist, 'No, no, this can't be true. You've made a mistake!'"

Even people with great self-confidence and strong fighting spirits may be daunted by cancer. "A diagnosis of cancer is . . . at a minimum . . . one of life's most dreaded personal crises" (Doan & Gray, 1992, p. 255). As LeShan (1989, p. 147) put it, "If you have cancer (or if someone you love has it), it is only rational to be sometimes irrational about it; to go a bit crazy from time to time."

Therapists can help by reassuring people that extreme distress, as well as depression and anxiety, are very understandable reactions to the diagnosis of cancer and are unlikely to impair their prognosis. Fawzy and colleagues (1993) found that people who survived malignant melanoma initially had higher distress than those who died from the disease during the time of the study. Researchers generally agree that short-lived distress and expression of negative emotions at the time of diagnosis are associated with a good prognosis (Dean & Hopwood, 1989). For most people, the initially high level of distress resolves itself within a few weeks, although distress will wax and wane throughout the treatment process (Massie & Holland, 1992).

Therapists can help people explore the meaning they ascribe to cancer, whether it is viewed as a challenge, a punishment, or a way to gain attention and let go of responsibilities. Bernie Siegel (1993), among others, advanced the belief that cancer often provides desired secondary gains. Although this is certainly not the case for all people with cancer, it is worth considering when trying to understand a person's experience with cancer.

Finding a meaning to the illness has been positively correlated with adjustment to the illness (Heim, 1991). People who attribute their disease to external causes (such as contagion, environment, chance, trauma) generally cope better than those who attribute cancer to internal factors (for example, heredity, punishment, constitutional susceptibility) or who have no explanation for the disease (Bearison, Sadow, Granowetter, & Winkel, 1993). This may be because people believe they can have the greatest control over external causes. Exploring the meaning a person has made of cancer will facilitate understanding of the kind of help that will be most useful to that person.

Sometimes the meaning will not seem logical to the therapist; however, attributing the disease to an understandable cause may provide a sense of control for the person with cancer. Even explanations that involve self-blame may be helpful in alleviating confusion and a sense of vulnerability. Therapists should be cautious about questioning the meaning people make of their disease.

Another common response to the diagnosis of cancer is to ask, "Why me?" This question seems to be associated with a perceived loss of control and a belief that something could have been done to prevent the cancer. This self-blaming attitude has been associated with a poorer adjustment to the diagnosis (Lowery, Jacobson, & DuCette, 1993).

Deciding who and how to tell about the diagnosis, mobilizing support systems along the way. Most people have many groups of friends and associates including nuclear family, family of origin, close and casual friends, business colleagues (supervisors, peers, employees), and neighbors. Deciding who to tell as well as how much and when to tell about their disease are important concerns for most cancer survivors. Being diagnosed with cancer is of course a very personal matter. Some people feel no discomfort in talking freely about their disease while others feel stigmatized or ashamed, especially if their cancer is such that they might be blamed for it (lung cancer in a person who smokes) or their appearance or functioning altered.

When people inform others of their disease is an opportune time to ask for help. Therapists can help clients plan how to communicate information about their disease to others and to define, as specifically as possible, what help they need and who can provide it.

Gathering information. Although several decades ago many people with cancer were not told of their diagnosis, physicians now would be viewed as unethical if they withheld such information. Beyond the diagnosis, however, the amount of information that medical staff share with cancer survivors varies widely, depending on the physician, the patient, the family, and their interrelationships. Borysenko (1988) argued for people to have full information; knowing when and what to anticipate can allay fears and help people to relax. Knowledge also promotes a sense of control. As Borysenko (1988, p. 22) stated, "People who feel in control of life can withstand an enormous amount of change."

During the first few weeks after diagnosis, cancer survivors typically feel confused and overwhelmed. They may feel inundated with new terms, choices, and possibilities. How much detailed information people desire varies: some want to read copies of their laboratory reports and research their disease while others prefer a general summary. Therapists should help people identify their comfort level and then help them to obtain the information they need to make sound decisions without feeling overwhelmed. Therapists can then help people to organize and process this information, to formulate and write down their questions, and to determine how to go about getting those answers.

Making and implementing decisions and plans. Physicians seem to encourage people with cancer to make treatment decisions rapidly. People need to ascertain how long they can wait to make a decision without undermining their prognosis. They can then break their decisions down into small, manageable steps and proceed to tackle them in a systematic way. A particularly difficult decision faced by many people with cancer is whether to become involved in clinical trials, studies of promising new treatments that may be more effective than standard treatments but that have not yet conclusively proven their value. If appropriate, people can be reminded that a physician is making a recommendation, not a decision; viewing that recommendation along with other information or opinions in combination with the person's preferences is likely to lead to the best decision for a particular individual.

Developing/maintaining a sense of self-efficacy and mastery. Zimpfer (1989) found that people who have been diagnosed with cancer typically experience losses in four important areas:

1. Loss of identity, due to increased dependence, physical changes.

2. Loss of control: they need to be cared for and no longer have control over their lives and time.

3. Loss of social support and contact.

4. Loss of time: uncertainty about the future, coupled with a sense of urgency about decisions.

All four of these losses may be experienced with the initial diagnosis of cancer and may persist throughout the treatment process.

Jacobson and Holland (1991) found that perceived control over both cancer and its side effects was negatively correlated with emotional distress. Obtaining information and taking charge of decision making are ways to gain a sense of competence and control and to address feelings of loss. LeShan (1989) suggested taking the perspective of what is right with a person rather than what is wrong, focusing on what gives the person a sense of enthusiasm and energy rather than on the disease. Helping people to identify and build on strengths and coping mechanisms they have used successfully in the past will help them cope with cancer. Emphasis should be on reasons to live. Coping mechanisms can be further developed as therapy progresses, but initially, old coping mechanisms need to be shored up and built on as quickly as possible.

Winograd (1992, p. 138) developed the following pledge for people with cancer. Reading this pledge aloud and keeping a copy of it for frequent review can be reassuring and empowering, especially during the early weeks of a cancer diagnosis:

I will be heard.

I will not be intimidated.

I will listen to my body; my symptoms matter.

I will be fully informed and be included in the final decision.

I will have the best care.

I am entitled to hope.

I am entitled to compassion and to be treated with dignity.

I will stand up for my own best interests.

I will praise good care and report bad care.

I will be safe.

A sense of competence and direction can be fostered not only by addressing the demands of the disease but also by helping people to live more deliberately in other areas of their lives. Deciding what to do each day, incorporating activities that are enjoyable and give a sense of accomplishment, can be empowering.

Treatment

Approximately one-third of all people with cancer do not comply fully with their recommended treatment regimens (Doka, 1993). This is usually due to the frightening and aversive nature of the treatments. Treatment compliance may be increased by helping people both to modify the treatments so that they are more acceptable and to deal more successfully with the potential side effects of the treatment.

Treatment is likely to be particularly difficult for people with early-stage cancers who were feeling well and may have had no apparent symptoms. Reactions of resistance and resentment often develop when the treatment makes them feel sicker than they felt before the diagnosis. Prophylactic treatment, such as radiation after apparently successful surgery for breast cancer, is also likely to evoke strong feelings of resistance.

Understanding the importance of their treatments and finding they can exert some control over them can help cancer survivors to accept those treatments. This does not mean that they are happy about or enjoy their treatments but rather, "Acceptance is realizing that to do *other* than accept is a) painful and b) futile" (McWilliams & McWilliams, 1991, p. 471). Having clear information on their treatments and their probable side effects also helps to promote acceptance by enabling people to plan and manage their lives more successfully. In addition, tailoring the treatment to each person's preferences as much as possible has resulted in better psychological adjustment (Leinster, Ashcroft, Slade, & Dewey, 1989). Even minor changes like scheduling radiotherapy at the end of the day so the person can spend most of the day at the office, allowing blood tests to be done by the technician of choice, and arranging for a private room for the person recovering from surgery can make an enormous difference in attitudes toward treatment.

Surgery and Hospitalization

The usual goal of surgery, for people with cancer, is to excise the cancer as well as a safe margin of surrounding tissue. Nearby lymph nodes, such as those under the arm for people with breast cancer, may also be removed as an index of whether the cancer has spread beyond the local site. Many aspects of surgery are frightening. The isolation and sterile environment of the hospital can cause discomfort. Anesthesia is a source of concern; some people fear they will not awaken from general anesthesia. If the surgery is for diagnostic purposes, the uncertainty may evoke high distress. Women undergoing biopsies to determine whether they had breast cancer, for example, had an average anxiety level that was comparable to that of people who had been hospitalized because of an acute anxiety reaction (Jacobson & Holland, 1991). Fear that a fatal or disfiguring error will be made in the process of surgery is common (Barraclough, 1994). Of course, the recovery from surgery may entail pain and discomfort as well as a convalescent period when usual activities must be curtailed. Finally, the surgery may result in prolonged or permanent bodily changes and loss of functioning. Particularly high levels of emotional disorders have been associated with what have been called mutilating surgeries (Hughes, 1987).

The surgery that has been most studied is mastectomy or removal of the breast following a diagnosis of breast cancer. Moorey and Greer (1989) found that 20 to 25 percent of people who had mastectomies were clinically depressed one year after surgery. An even higher incidence of psychological problems was found in people who had colostomies. Depression as well as work-related problems were also common in people whose ability to speak was adversely affected by laryngectomies.

Matthews and Ridgeway (1984) identified six avenues to helping people prepare for surgery:

1. Procedural information: What will happen before, during, and after surgery?

2. Sensation information: What physical sensations such as pain or numbness are people likely to experience from surgery?

3. Behavioral instructions: What can people do to facilitate their recovery from surgery?

4. Modeling: Use of films, stories, or role models to prepare people for surgery, especially useful for children.

5. Relaxation: Procedures such as meditation, hypnosis, deep breathing, and imagery to help people control surgery-related anxiety.

6. Cognitive skills: Techniques such as affirmations and positive self-talk can help people view surgery in a different light.

People seem to cope more successfully with surgery if they have a clear understanding of the anticipated nature and impact of the surgery and of methods that are available to help them regain their normal functioning and appearance as soon as and as much as possible. In addition, once people have this information, they can then make decisions and request procedures that will help them.

The indignity and depersonalization often connected to surgical procedures can be particularly upsetting. Reviewing with people the information they have been given about their upcoming surgeries can lead to identification of areas likely to raise anxiety so that ways to address those areas can be developed. One woman, for example, felt dehumanized by being wheeled into the surgery room; she persuaded her physician to allow her to walk into the surgery room on her own. Another person who had read about the importance of subliminal messages during surgery asked her doctors to make only positive comments and healing statements during the surgical procedure and to play tapes of music she used for relaxation. A third person wanted to wear his wedding ring while undergoing surgery. Arrangements were made for him to do so. Even minor accommodations like these can give a sense of control and reassurance to someone about to undergo surgery.

A particularly important issue is receiving information. Biopsies and other surgical procedures provide important information on a person's diagnosis and prognosis. Physicians have been known to give people negative information while they are still confused and groggy from the anesthesia. The patient, along with close family members, should be encouraged to decide when and to whom diagnostic information should be given to ensure that cancer survivors are not given information when they are likely to feel vulnerable and alone. People who anticipate surgery also can benefit from deciding what support systems they want to have available and asking family and friends to be with them before and after the surgery.

Chemotherapy

Chemotherapy is a treatment for certain cancers including leukemias, lymphomas, testicular tumors, breast cancer, and some types of lung cancer. Chemotherapy generally is combined with

surgery or radiation when cancerous lymph nodes or other indications of regional disease spread are present (Jacobson & Holland,
1991). Chemotherapy involves treatment with one or a combination of very powerful, cytotoxic drugs that can kill the cancer cells.
In the process, of course, normal cells, particularly those that are
rapidly dividing as in the intestinal lining and in hair follicles, are
also damaged. Side effects of chemotherapy including hair loss, nausea and vomiting, mouth sores, fatigue and depression, discolored
nails, constipation and diarrhea, and susceptibility to infection, and
many others are common. The number of chemotherapy side effects
that a person experiences is more strongly correlated with level of
distress than is the severity of the side effects (Jacobson & Holland,
1991). Particularly difficult times for most people receiving
chemotherapy are before the first treatment; midway through a
series of treatments; the few days before and after each treatment
when nausea is most likely; and seven to ten days after a treatment
when blood counts are most affected.

The side effects of chemotherapy are severe enough to cause
many people to halt their treatment before it is completed. Consequently, helping people cope with these side effects can make a
great difference in their prognosis. Distress associated with the side
effects of chemotherapy can be reduced through effective coping
and control over those side effects.

The use of chemotherapy as a preventive or adjuvant measure
has increased in recent years, particularly in the treatment of breast
cancer. Studies have shown that even for people with early-stage
breast cancer, chemotherapy can reduce the likelihood of a metastasis or spread of the cancer. People receiving prophylactic
chemotherapy seem to have a particularly difficult time with the
process (Moorey & Greer, 1989). They may view the treatment as
optional and possibly unnecessary and do not seem to have the
same motivation toward treatment as people who know the
chemotherapy is needed to save their lives. Particularly for people
who otherwise feel well, chemotherapy may be resented because in

the short run it is making them ill rather than healthy and because during the months of treatment, they have a continual reminder of their disease, a disruption that probably makes it difficult for them to resume their normal activities.

Chemotherapy usually entails a series of treatments in which the drugs are administered intravenously in an outpatient setting. Although for some cancers there has been a trend toward fewer administrations of more powerful drugs, multiple sessions of chemotherapy are the norm. These may be relatively brief or may be prolonged for drugs that must be infused into the system slowly in order to control their toxic impact. This pattern of repeat visits often conditions people undergoing chemotherapy to develop phobic reactions to the treatment. Redd (1988) found that 25 to 65 percent of people undergoing chemotherapy developed emotional or behavioral difficulties in response to treatment, most commonly anxiety and insomnia prior to treatments and anticipatory nausea and vomiting associated with the administration of highly emetic drugs.

Anticipatory nausea (AN), defined as nausea that occurs before a chemotherapy treatment, is experienced by 18 to 57 percent of people undergoing chemotherapy while 9 to 33 percent have anticipatory vomiting (Andrykowski & Jacobson, 1993). These reactions are associated with a history of emotional instability and of motion sickness, an expectation of experiencing nausea, and with current distress and anxiety, as well as with the number of chemotherapy treatments and the severity of the vomiting induced by those treatments (Andrykowski & Jacobson, 1993; Hursti et al., 1992). AN can be triggered by any reminder of the chemotherapy, the building, the physician, a sound or smell, or even the knowledge that chemotherapy is imminent. This can be generalized to other settings and can be very troubling, usually worsening over the course of chemotherapy unless help is provided. One person receiving chemotherapy became nauseated whenever she went to the airport because the heating system created an odor she associated with the medical clinic where she received her chemotherapy. Family and friends may erroneously view AN as a sign of weaknesses, thereby worsening the situation by contributing to the cancer survivor's self-doubts and interpersonal difficulties.

Cognitive-Behavioral Approaches to Facilitate Chemotherapy

Cognitive-behavioral procedures have been found effective in ameliorating negative reactions to chemotherapy.

Relaxation training. Relaxation, induced via deep breathing, progressive muscle relaxation, meditation, music, biofeedback, or hypnosis, and coupled with a pleasant scene, has been shown to produce significant reductions in the duration, intensity, and frequency of anticipatory nausea (Redd, 1988). Carey and Burish (1987) set up an experimental study of relaxation training with people undergoing chemotherapy. Their study had four treatment conditions: (1) progressive muscle relaxation training and guided imagery delivered by professional therapists, (2) the same training done by trained volunteers and paraprofessional therapists, (3) the same training delivered via audiotapes, and (4) antiemetic medication only. The training began with a forty-five-minute session prior to the first chemotherapy administration. People were instructed to practice the techniques at home. Those in group 1 had significantly greater reductions in anxiety and physiological arousal as well as increased food intake compared with the other three groups.

Systematic desensitization. In this three-step process, a hierarchy of anxiety-provoking stimuli is first developed. This list might begin with making the appointment for the chemotherapy treatment, creating a low level of anxiety; proceed through stimuli such as driving to the clinic, parking in the lot, walking into the building, and signing in, all creating moderate levels of anxiety; and finally sitting in the special chair, seeing the chemotherapy drugs being readied, and receiving the chemotherapy, all creating high levels of anxiety. Once the list has been developed, therapists help clients visualize each situation while in a calm, relaxed state, starting with the least aversive image. Suggestions of a sense of competence and empowerment can accelerate the process. Movement from one visualization to the next occurs only when the person feels comfortable and in control in each situation. This process has been shown to result in less severe and briefer periods of AN (Redd, 1988).

Distraction. Focusing attention on positive stimuli can successfully block the impact of negative stimuli. For example, Redd et al. (1987) made video games available prior to chemotherapy to people between the ages of nine and twenty. The distraction provided by the video games resulted in significantly less nausea as well as some reduction in self-reported anxiety.

Hypnotherapy and suggestion. A controlled study of interventions for chemotherapy distress in children found that hypnosis involving imaginative fantasies before and during chemotherapy, coupled with suggestions of security, feeling good, feeling hungry, and wanting to socialize was even more powerful than cognitive distraction (jokes, magic tricks) and relaxation in relieving anticipatory and postchemotherapy nausea. People who received cognitive distraction or relaxation did experience some improvement in nausea levels, however, while those in the control group who received only conversation with a therapist showed an increase in symptoms (Zeltzer, Dolgin, Le Baron, & Le Baron, 1991).

Positive motivation. Pairing each chemotherapy session with a reward or positive reinforcement can take away some of its aversive impact. For children, the reward may be a special privilege or treat. Adults too can use this approach by rewarding themselves with a special activity or purchase such as a good mystery novel to read while recovering from chemotherapy. The reward can provide a bright spot in an otherwise unpleasant activity.

Modeling through imagery. Another approach that has been effective in reducing negative reactions to chemotherapy in children and adolescents is telling stories about their favorite heroes coping with chemotherapy and other aversive medical procedures. The storyteller can gradually increase the realism in the stories until it approximates the situation the child is experiencing. Positive identification with the hero's behavior can motivate and empower the young person. Adults can use a variation on this technique. By acting as if they are an admired athlete, film star, friend, or colleague, they can gain a greater sense of competence and control.

Cognitive restructuring and affirmations. Changing what people tell themselves about chemotherapy also can make a difference in the severity of their side effects. The person who repeats, "One more down, only two more to go; I can do it" to himself or herself is likely to feel better than the person who says, "That last chemotherapy session was awful. How can I stand another one? I'll never get through all my treatments."

Environmental manipulation. Providing an orientation session to people about to undergo chemotherapy can be helpful. A ninety-minute session with the patient and family members scheduled before the first chemotherapy session, including a tour of the oncology site, a videotape of someone coping effectively with chemotherapy, training in relaxation and imagery, and an opportunity to receive answers to questions, was associated with a reduction in anticipatory side effects and negative affect, improved overall coping, and less disruption of activities (Burish, Snyder, & Jenkins, 1991).

Changing the conditions of the chemotherapy also can be helpful. Scheduling the treatment for the first appointment in the morning can eliminate hours of anxiety, minimize uncomfortable time spent in the waiting room, and avoid exposure to other people having chemotherapy. Mints or other strong tastes or smells paired with chemotherapy can mask sensations associated with chemotherapy that may trigger AN. (This approach does have the risk of linking negative experiences to otherwise benign tastes or smells.) Having a friend or relative accompany a cancer survivor to the treatment to provide support, distraction, and an opportunity to express feelings also can be helpful. Research found that people who had a companion with them when they received information on chemotherapy maintained higher self-esteem and a greater sense of well-being than those who received the information alone (Ward, Leventhal, Easterling, Luchterhand, & Love, 1991).

Antiemetic medication such as Ziphrain as well as antianxiety medication has also been helpful in reducing both anticipatory and reactive nausea and vomiting associated with chemotherapy. Antiemetics seem to work best when used prophylactically rather than on an as needed basis (Andrykowski & Jacobson, 1993). However, these drugs also have their own side effects. Antiemetic medication, for example, can cause restlessness and agitation (Fleishman, Lesko, & Breitbart, 1993). Therapists might help cancer survivors decide whether medication for the side effects of chemotherapy offers more benefits than difficulties.

Dietary changes, such as the presentation of small, interesting meals in a relaxing setting, can help counteract the diminished appetite and weight loss that often results from nausea and mouth sores related to chemotherapy. Accurate information on the nature of the chemotherapy side effects can also be reassuring. Cancer survivors sometimes attribute symptoms to a worsening of their disease and need to know what symptoms are simply an unpleasant reaction to chemotherapy.

Overview of Interventions for Chemotherapy Side Effects

Although psychotherapy to help people cope with chemotherapy need not be prolonged, it seems most effective if it is multifaceted, begins before the first chemotherapy treatment, uses cognitive-behavioral techniques, involves practice of skills at home between sessions, involves friends or family members, and conveys feelings of control, empowerment, and self-efficacy.

Anxiety at the End of Chemotherapy

According to Susan Love, noted authority on breast cancer and its treatment, "The hardest time psychologically is after the treatments are completed" (Wadler, 1992, p. 179). Although nearly everyone undergoing chemotherapy eagerly anticipates its conclusion, they are often surprised to find their anxiety increasing once it is over. When people are receiving chemotherapy on a regular basis, they have close contact with their medical team; that contact, coupled with the chemotherapy, reassures them that everything possible is being done to cure their disease. However, once the treatments are over, they may miss the support of that "umbrella of protection" (Haber, 1993, p. 33). Therapists can ameliorate this reaction by warning cancer survivors that it is common, normalizing it if it does occur, allowing people an opportunity to express their anxiety, and helping them use cognitive-behavioral skills (discussed in Chapters Five and Six) as well as communication with their treatment team to cope with the anxiety.

Radiotherapy

Many types of radiation treatment are available. External beam radiation, in which a machine delivers X rays directly to the site of the tumor, is the most common type used to treat cancer (Winograd, 1992).

Although cancer survivors seem to dread surgery and chemotherapy more than they do radiotherapy or radiation treatment, radiation too presents difficulties. The numerous, frequent treatments can interfere with other responsibilities. The experience of being alone in a darkened room, partially dressed, and knowing that one is receiving a treatment that itself is potentially a carcinogen can be disconcerting. Fatigue as well as burning of the skin where the radiation is focused are common unpleasant side effects. Other side effects such as scarring, nausea, or hair loss may or may not be present, depending on the part of the body that receives the radiation. Psychological symptoms that have been associated with radiotherapy include lethargy, withdrawal, agitation, anxiety, hostility, a sense of isolation and discouragement (Jacobson & Holland, 1991; Moorey & Greer, 1989).

Preparation for radiotherapy and the radiotherapy itself may cause discomfort. Prior to the treatment, cancer survivors will usu-

ally be assessed by a medical team including a radiation oncologist
and a dosimetrist who will determine the exact dosage, schedule,
and placement of the radiation. To ensure accuracy, the cancer survivor may be tattooed with some tiny dots to mark the location that
is to be radiated. This may entail several hours of lying on a table,
partially clothed, while a group of people take measurements and
discuss the treatment. This can be a dehumanizing and uncomfortable experience, particularly if it comes as a surprise.

The delivery of the radiotherapy too may cause discomfort. Can
cer survivors will be alone in the treatment room, while the technician administers the treatment from a safe location, perhaps
observing through a window. For many, this creates a feeling of personal violation. In addition, the placement of the technician behind
insulated walls serves as a reminder of the potential danger inherent in radiation; it can contribute to the development of one cancer
while it is curing another.

Perhaps the most difficult aspect of radiotherapy is the impact it
has on a person's life. Radiotherapy typically is scheduled five days
a week for four to five weeks. For a month or more, people receiving this treatment must adapt their schedules to allow time for
transportation to and from the treatment facility as well as time for
the treatment. This demanding schedule, combined with the usual
fatigue that results from radiotherapy, may make it difficult if not
impossible for people to return to work or maintain other usual
activities. In addition, treatment that may be prophylactic is a constant and perhaps upsetting reminder that the person has been diagnosed with a potentially life-threatening disease.

Psychotherapy can help people deal more effectively with radiotherapy. Forester, Kornfeld, and Fleiss (1985) found that individual
psychotherapy that was supportive, educational, interpretive, and
cathartic led to alleviation of emotional symptoms (depression, pessimism, anxiety) as well as physical symptoms (loss of appetite,
fatigue, nausea, vomiting) associated with radiotherapy. Decker,
Cline-Elsen, and Gallagher (1992) studied the impact of relaxation,

including progressive muscle relaxation, deep breathing, and cued relaxation (pairing the word *calm* with a relaxed state), on people undergoing radiotherapy. People in the experimental condition met in small groups for six one-hour sessions and were given taped and written instructions to facilitate practice between sessions. People in the treatment condition showed a reduction in tension, anger, and depression while those in the control group experienced worsening of depression and fatigue. Whether the key ingredients were the group support, the relaxation techniques, or some combination of the two cannot be determined from this study.

Although more research is needed on the use of psychotherapy with people who are receiving radiotherapy, research suggests that the use of such techniques as information giving, exploration of feelings, relaxation, meditation, mental imagery, and cognitive restructuring may be very helpful to them. Both individual and group approaches to treatment seem effective and once again a multifaceted approach seems most beneficial.

Other Aversive Procedures

In addition to surgery, chemotherapy, and radiotherapy, cancer survivors may undergo a variety of other procedures. These procedures include those that may cause emotional distress but are not physically uncomfortable (X rays, bone scans), those that may be somewhat physically uncomfortable as well emotionally distressing (computed tomography or CT scans that entail drinking a large quantity of chalky fluid; multiple blood tests; and magnetic resonance imaging or MRI in which the person is surrounded by a tube-like apparatus during the testing), and those that have a profound physical and emotional impact (bone marrow aspirations, bone marrow transplantation).

Bone Marrow Transplantation

Bone marrow transplantation (BMT), used for treatment of leukemia and metastatic breast cancer as well as for other forms of cancer, is perhaps the most difficult of these procedures. It can entail 40 to 100 days in the hospital, often geographically removed from support systems, as well as severe limitations on activities for another six to twelve months. One study of people who had a BMT at least six months earlier found that more than 25 percent continued to focus primarily on the losses they had sustained from the procedure (Curbow, Legro, Baker, Wingard, & Somerfield, 1993). Adjustment was affected by many factors including the cancer survivors' developmental stage, the nature of their disease, their prior levels of adjustment, cultural and religious attitudes, support systems, their personality and coping styles, and their potential for rehabilitation. Those who could find a meaning in their disease and its treatment, perhaps a new perspective on their lives, new goals, or improved family relationships, were particularly likely to adjust well to the procedure. In light of this, psychotherapy with an existential emphasis may be appropriate for people facing BMTs.

Magnetic Resonance Imaging

Although MRI is certainly a less aversive procedure, approximately 20 percent of cancer survivors develop anxiety severe enough to interfere with the completion of an MRI scan. During the MRI, the person's body may be closely surrounded by a tube, a highly detailed diagnostic device that portrays the body's soft, internal tissues. Loud, jarring noises may occur repeatedly during the procedure. Such techniques as soothing music, muscle relaxation, paced breathing, and meditation can prevent or relieve the claustrophobic sensations that often develop during the procedure.

Venipuncture and Other Aversive Procedures

Venipuncture for blood tests as well as such aversive procedures as bone marrow aspirations and lumbar punctures can be especially difficult for children with cancer as well as for their parents. Carpenter (1991) found that children younger than seven experienced five to ten times the distress that older children experienced in response to such invasive procedures. Up to a third of cancer survivors between the ages of three and nine must be held down during these procedures. This is very difficult for the parents who often are present to offer support.

Carpenter (1991) found that children who perceived that they had some control over the procedures were less distressed than those who reported having no control. Giving the child choices such as which arm to use for a blood test or whether to get the test before or after lunch, as well as other approaches to promote a sense of control, are therefore important.

Hypnotherapy is another approach that has been found useful with children experiencing fear of medical procedures (Redd, 1988). Children generally are easier to hypnotize than adults and can readily be taught to focus on thoughts or images unrelated to pain they are experiencing. This approach is particularly effective with children who have the capacity to engage in fantasy and who become deeply involved in reading.

Four additional techniques have been found likely to reduce distress for children undergoing venipuncture as well as for their parents (Manne et al., 1990):

1. *Attentional distraction*. Party blowers were used to distract children in the above study.

2. *Substitution of incompatible positive responses for an undesirable behavior*. Desired behaviors were reinforced, positive self-talk was encouraged, and paced breathing, deep muscle relaxation, and imagery were used successfully to promote relaxation during difficult medical treatments.

3. *Positive reinforcement*. Stickers were given when children completed an aversive procedure. Filmed modeling of cooperative behavior was also used.

4. *Parental involvement*. Parents were encouraged to use distraction with their children as well as to count to set the pace for the children's breathing.

Although the children in the above studies continued to report pain, their observed distress and pain reactions were reduced as was parental anxiety.

Physical Changes Associated with Cancer

Cancer and its treatment can cause both short-term, temporary physical changes and long-term, enduring or permanent physical changes. Common short-term changes include alterations in taste and smell, weight change, difficulty sleeping, fatigue, oral ulcerations (mouth sores), hair loss, changes in the color of the skin and nails, itching, hemorrhoids, constipation or diarrhea, and many other less common symptoms. These changes can contribute to the depression and anxiety cancer survivors may already be experiencing, damage self-esteem and self-efficacy, and further complicate the difficult process of coping with cancer. Role changes, due to lost time at work or inability to maintain one's usual schedule of personal and professional responsibilities, can also cause distress and a sense of losing one's place in life.

Therapists should spend time exploring with cancer survivors what physical changes they are experiencing and how they are affected by and coping with those changes. What may seem to some like a minor inconvenience when there is the possibility of dying from cancer may be very significant to others. One cancer survivor, for example, elected not to have the recommended chemotherapy because it would result in hair loss, even though it would improve her prognosis.

Although psychotherapy cannot eliminate most of the side effects of cancer treatments, it may be able to reduce the severity of some of them, such as eating and sleeping difficulties, and the distress associated with all of them. Approaches discussed earlier in this chapter as well as in Chapters Five and Six of this book—relaxation, mental imagery, hypnotherapy, cognitive restructuring, and affirmations—can all be used to help people cope with the short-term impact of cancer. Practical accommodations, such as an attractive wig purchased before chemotherapy begins or schedule changes to allow time for naps and multiple small meals, also can promote effective coping with these changes. In addition, support and empathy from family, friends, and other cancer survivors who are dealing with the same changes, as well as an opportunity to express feelings and examine choices in a structured, organized way, can help. Also helpful are viewing the side effects as a temporary part of the process of treatment and rewards such as a vacation when the person's strength is adequate and a new outfit when some weight has been regained.

Long-Term Physical Changes Associated with Cancer Treatments

In recent years, advances in surgical procedures for people with cancer have led to less extensive surgery, especially in treating breast cancer and cancers in the limbs. Nevertheless, cancer treatment often does cause permanent physical changes. Significant physical changes due to cancer and its treatment may include loss of part of the body (a breast or a limb), loss of an important ability (vision, speech), or loss of future possibilities (infertility due to radiotherapy or chemotherapy-induced menopause, loss of occupation due to intellectual changes).

An altered body image can be devastating to one's self-esteem as can associated loss of important roles and activities. Edgar, Rosberger, and Nowlis (1992) found, for example, that 33 percent of people who had undergone mastectomies continued to experience severe emotional distress two years after their surgery. People who experience facial disfigurement as a result of head and neck cancer have a very high incidence of clinical depression and suicidal ideation (Mellette, 1989). High emotional distress, including fear of rejection and abandonment, also is common in people who have lost the capacity for normal speech due to a laryngectomy (Dropkin, 1990).

Goals for therapists helping people deal with significant physical changes due to cancer usually include promoting as much recovery of functioning as possible, reducing psychological distress and maintaining good self-esteem, and maximizing quality of life. Psychotherapists have several approaches available to help people deal with these physical changes:

Expressing emotions and grief work. Betty Rollin (1976) wrote *First You Cry* about her diagnosis of breast cancer and her subsequent mastectomy. The expression of those strong feelings of sorrow and grief that almost inevitably accompany a major physical loss is the first step. This is a process that takes time, much like mourning a death, and may be reawakened by painful reminders of the change, an anniversary, an activity that must be given up, an outfit that can no longer be worn.

Cognitive-behavioral psychotherapy. Cognitive approaches can help people put the physical changes in perspective and appreciate the possible benefit their treatments have brought them in improving their health. Therapists should be careful not to minimize a loss but rather to encourage cancer survivors to reframe their losses in ways that are meaningful to them. Only the cancer survivor can say, "Losing my breast was dreadful, but it could have been worse, I could have lost a leg or an arm" or "I lost one eye but I still have another one."

Behavioral approaches are especially useful at helping cancer survivors maximize their activity levels. Holley (1983), for example, found that psychotherapy was successful in motivating people to learn esophageal speech after they had a laryngectomy. Without help, as many as a third do not acquire this speech (Stam, Koopmans, & Mathieson, 1991). Modeling by other cancer survivors is a particularly helpful intervention. Hospital visits by "fellow laryngectomees" was associated with a subsequently better quality of life in people who had that surgery (Stam, Koopmans, & Mathieson, 1991). Also, a program called Reach to Recovery has had good results from having breast cancer survivors visit people in the hospital who have recently undergone surgery for breast cancer.

Surgery as well as chemotherapy and radiotherapy typically curtail a person's activities. Resuming rewarding roles and activities, as well as developing new ones, can reduce depression and help cancer survivors recognize that their lives can still be rewarding despite the changes they have experienced.

Rehabilitation and reconstruction. These procedures can help cancer survivors to regain as much of their former capacities and appearance as possible. Physical therapy can develop skills and strengths to compensate for those that have been lost. Reconstruction is widely used for people who have mastectomies and can even be done concurrent with the mastectomy so the person is never without a breast. Choosing to have breast reconstruction has been found to be a sign of mental health and to promote improved adjustment (Redd & Jacobson, 1988). Prosthetic devices also can be used to improve appearance when surgery is not feasible. Therapists can help their clients to explore these options and decide what is best for them.

Family counseling. Family members and close friends also have reactions to the losses and changes and their reactions can color those of the cancer survivor. One woman's husband, for example, reacted to her mastectomy scar by saying, "Boy, they sure messed you up." From that point on, she refused to let him see her unclothed and withdrew sexually. Feelings of revulsion, as well as fear of physically hurting the cancer survivor, are sometimes reported by family members providing care for people who have had tracheostomies or colostomies (Shapiro & Kornfeld, 1987). Helping close family and friends to process their own reactions, to have their feelings accepted and understood, to appreciate the potential impact of those reactions on cancer survivors, and to promote dialogue between survivor and friend or family member can facilitate adjustment to a loss.

Participation in a support group. National and local support groups are available for people with all of the major types of cancer. Some of these are listed in the Resources section at the end of this book.

Sharing feelings, learning skills from each other, and having the role models provided by such groups can contribute a great deal to reducing depression, isolation, and feelings of loss experienced by people who have significant physical changes due to cancer treatments.

Awareness of legal rights. Cancer survivors whose treatment resulted in a physical or mental impairment that limits their work activities may well be protected by legislation. In 1986, a resolution was passed unanimously by both the United States Senate and House of Representatives, expressing the opposition of Congress to employment discrimination against people who have or have had cancer (Mellette, 1989). The Federal Rehabilitation Act of 1973 bans employment discrimination based on disabilities by employers that receive federal funds. Other legislation prohibits employment discrimination against people with disabilities by private employers and requires employers to make reasonable accommodation to the needs of disabled workers. These regulations are enforced by the Equal Employment Opportunities Commission. Therapists who assume an advocacy role can help their clients become aware of and safeguard their rights.

Cancer-Related Changes in Sexuality and Fertility

One of the most common and unfortunate changes caused by cancer and its treatment is impairment in sexual and reproductive capacity. Hughes (1987) found that 50 percent of cancer survivors reported a diminution in sexual interest and 10 to 20 percent reported severe sexual dysfunction. According to Moorey and Greer (1989), "There is documented evidence of impaired sexual functioning in a substantial proportion of patients with cancers of the breast, bowel, female genital tract, prostate, and testis" (p. 166). Chemotherapy and hormone treatment can cause premature menopause, along with decreased arousal and painful intercourse. Radiation to the reproductive organs can cause permanent sterility.

Surgery for prostate cancer may cause temporary or even permanent sexual dysfunction (although recent medical advances have reduced the likelihood of that side effect). All aspects of the sexual response cycle—desire, excitement, and orgasm—can be impaired by cancer and its treatment.

In addition, "cancer does not have to involve sexual organs to affect sexual functioning. All cancers affect body image and self-image and thus have the potential to diminish sexual functioning, especially with regard to feelings of sexual attractiveness" (Burbie & Polinsky, 1992, p. 20). Bodily changes due to mastectomies and other surgeries can cause cancer survivors to view themselves as undesirable and unattractive and to avoid intimate contact. Kaplan (1992) reported that women being treated for breast cancer often seemed more fearful of losing their intimate partners than they were of the prospect of death. Usually, this fear of relationships ending in response to cancer is unfounded, but the fear itself can lead to sexual avoidance in anticipation of rejection.

In addition, survival concerns may seem so overwhelming that cancer survivors in the midst of treatment may have little energy or interest left over for intimacy. Depression commonly reduces sexual desire. Of course, so does the fatigue and nausea accompanying chemotherapy.

The partners may contribute to these difficulties by viewing the cancer survivors as less attractive and also may avoid physical contact out of a fear of touching or injuring treated areas of the body. Partners even may fear that cancer can be transmitted through sexual activity (Barraclough, 1994). Both partner and survivor may be reluctant to initiate sexual activity; avoidance and feelings of rejection may escalate on both sides. In addition, for people who want to have children, loss of fertility may seem to have dashed their hopes for a happy future.

Unfortunately, according to Helen Singer Kaplan (1992, p. 3), the sexual side effects of cancer treatment have "been largely neglected by researchers, oncologists, and surgeons, as well as by mental health specialists." Psychotherapists should be sure to inquire about cancer survivors' sexual feelings and behaviors during and after treatment and any changes that may have ensued in functioning, enjoyment, and fertility. Unless this discussion is initiated by the therapist, these issues may be avoided or ignored. The survivors may be embarrassed to bring up these issues or may view them as relatively unimportant in the face of the life-or-death issues they are confronting.

Schover, Evans, and von Eschenbach (1987) found that extended, intensive rather than brief treatment generally was necessary to reverse sexual dysfunction in cancer survivors. Psychotherapy seems to be most effective if it involves both the survivor and the partner and if counseling is used preventively, beginning as soon as treatment is planned that may have a negative impact on sexual image and functioning (Schover & Fife, 1986). Goals for psychotherapy with cancer survivors who have suffered sexual and fertility changes usually are similar to those discussed in the previous section and include the following:

• *Providing opportunity to explore and express feelings as well as to grieve physical losses and lost possibilities.*

• *Identifying ways to reduce the severity of the changes and their consequences.* Medical interventions may be available that will make a difference. For example, Cullinan (1992) found that for women who had breast cancer, the more radical the surgery, the greater the impact on the sexual and marital relationship. Women who had reconstructive breast surgery showed less sexual impairment than women who had lumpectomies (removal of a segment of the breast), who showed less impairment than women who had mastectomies (removal of the entire breast) without reconstruction. However, as long as eight years after their diagnosis, 50 percent of women who had had treatment for breast cancer continued to have sexual difficulties (Burbie & Polinsky, 1992). Kaplan (1992) found that testosterone was helpful to survivors of breast and other gynecological cancers who could not take estrogen because it might contribute to a recurrence.

Procedures are also available to help men who are threatened with loss of their reproductive capacity due to cancer treatments. Men may have their sperm frozen prior to their treatments so that it can be used later to inseminate their partners.

For useful information on medical treatment to address sexual issues, cancer survivors usually will have to consult not only their oncologists but also gynecologists, urologists, and other specialists. This is an area in which information seems limited and difficult to obtain and therapists may need to help cancer survivors assert themselves and cope with their embarrassment about asking physicians for help with sexual difficulties.

• *Promoting clear, open, and supportive communication between cancer survivors and their partners and encouraging resumption of sexual activity as soon as medically feasible* (Moorey & Greer, 1989). Some difficulties may be easily overcome by eliminating misunderstanding and initiating dialogue on difficult subjects. For other concerns, adaptation to changes and special needs may improve sexual functioning. Preexisting sexual and marital difficulties may be exacerbated by cancer treatments and those areas too may need attention.

• *Restoring or maintaining self-esteem and a rewarding quality of life that includes as satisfying a sexual relationship as the person wants to have and is capable of having.*

Reducing Pain

Perhaps the most feared and difficult consequence of cancer is pain. Pain may result from the cancer itself or from its treatment. Moderate to severe disease-related pain is experienced by 6 to 20 percent of people with nonmetastatic (early-stage) cancer, by 40 percent of adults in the intermediate stages of cancer, and by 60 to 90 percent in the advanced stages (Jay & Elliott, 1986; McGuire,

1987). Uncontrolled pain can lead to other difficulties such as sleeping problems, loss of appetite, anxiety, and depression. Among people with cancer, 39 percent of those with a mental disorder experienced significant pain while only 19 percent of those without a mental disorder had significant pain (Massie & Holland, 1992), suggesting that pain may cause considerable emotional dysfunction. Uncontrolled pain is also associated with greater risk for suicide. Relief of pain often results in the disappearance of a perceived psychiatric disorder (Breitbart & Passik, 1993). Although most cancer-related pain can be controlled by medication, cancer survivors may need help in requesting medication for pain relief and may benefit from a combination of medication and psychotherapy to reduce pain.

Psychotherapy has been shown to be as effective in reducing cancer-related pain as it has in ameliorating many of the other negative consequences of cancer and its treatment. Usual goals of psychotherapy for pain include providing support, information on cancer pain and its treatment, and skills that are likely to ameliorate the pain. Individual, group, and family therapy all have been found effective in helping people to manage cancer pain (Breitbart, 1989).

A gradual reduction in pain is usually a more realistic and less discouraging goal than elimination of the pain. A written or verbal rating scale of the severity of the pain is useful for both therapists and survivors to track the progress of their efforts. Breitbart and Passik (1993) suggested use of a visual analog scale of 0-10 for rating pain. (See Chapter Three for more information on this scale.) Physicians should be consulted before pain-reduction efforts are initiated to determine the cancer survivor's capacities and to ensure that reducing the pain will not sacrifice important medical information.

People with pain typically become passive and inactive, focusing their attention on the pain. This stance can worsen the pain. Teaching people a range of approaches to distract themselves, increase their activity levels as much as they are physically able, and transform the sensation of the pain can contribute to a reduction in discomfort. These techniques also can be used to prepare people to deal with painful medical procedures; in psychotherapy sessions, they can practice the techniques while imagining themselves undergoing the procedure.

Using Imagery

Imagery is one of the most powerful tools available to reduce pain. It can promote an alteration of sensations and can be used in any situation. Horowitz and Breitbart (1993) identified three approaches to using imagery for alleviation of cancer-related pain:

1. *Pleasant distracting imagery.* By envisioning themselves in a calm, restful scene or engaged in rewarding activities, cancer survivors can take their minds off the pain and reduce their perception of its severity. This can be especially effective for mild to moderate pain and for people who want to avoid or deny the severity of their condition, but this approach may be less effective for people who want to be fully informed and aware of what is happening to them (Golden, Gersh, & Robbins, 1992).

2. *Transformational imagery.* This approach uses guided imagery to change a person's experience of pain. It may be imagined as another sensation such as warmth, tingling, icy cold numbness, or pressure. This change can be facilitated through actual use of an ice pack or warm bath. The imagined size and shape of the pain also may be altered. The person might imagine expelling the pain with every breath. Changing the context of the pain may be helpful. Breitbart (1989) suggested imagining oneself on a battlefield with the pain resulting from a wound. Another approach is visualizing the pain as a creature and having an imaginary dialogue with the creature, asking what can be done to reduce the pain (Simonton, Matthews-Simonton, & Creighton, 1992).

3. *Dissociative imagery.* In this approach, people disconnect or dissociate themselves from the pain. This may be accomplished by their imagining themselves leaving their body and being pain-free or dissociating themselves from the painful part of their body.

Using Hypnosis

Hypnosis, an even more powerful form of imagery, also can be helpful to those people who are at least moderately hypnotizable. Foley (1986) found that 50 percent of cancer survivors could obtain pain relief from hypnosis. Spiegel (1985) recommended three principles to guide the use of hypnosis for pain: (1) filter the hurt out of the pain, (2) don't fight the pain, and (3) increase control. Like imagery, hypnosis can be used to anesthetize a part of the body or to create a change in sensation such as a temperature change or analgesia (dulling). Spiegel suggested asking whether warmth or cold will feel better and then inducing that sensation. Because pain and temperature fibers run together in the body, this can ameliorate pain. A mental filter may be imagined to ease the pain. For experienced hypnotherapists with highly hypnotizable clients, the use of age regression can relieve pain by taking people to a time when they were free of pain.

Using Cognitive-Behavioral Approaches

Because pain may be exacerbated by tension, relaxation techniques, especially those that are passive, such as focusing on breathing, can reduce pain through distraction and release of tension. Electromyographic and temperature biofeedback can be used in a similar way, to distract, promote control over the pain, and increase relaxation.

Other cognitive-behavioral techniques may also be helpful. According to Breitbart and Passik (1993, p. 51), "Beliefs about the meaning of pain and the presence of a mood disturbance are better predictors of level of pain than is the site of metastasis." Pain may be experienced as more severe and upsetting if it is believed to be a sign of the cancer progressing. Cognitive restructuring, particularly if based on encouraging medical information, can reduce pain. Other cognitive techniques such as affirmations, thought stopping, and letting thoughts drift through the mind may also be useful.

Behavioral interventions, designed to increase activity level (if medically advisable) and occupy attention, can also contribute to pain relief. For children, reinforcement of coping behaviors via toys or privileges can be very helpful as can imagining themselves as super heroes who can tolerate even severe pain. For cancer survivors of all ages, even quiet activities such as music or reading can calm and distract.

Using Other Strategies

Techniques such as information giving, support, opportunity to express feelings, and communication skills training, focused on asking for help with pain in a clear, calm way, can also be helpful. Pain also may be related to past experiences. Breitbart and Passik (1993) observed that the cancer setting could reawaken traumatic memories and that pain could be a dissociative symptom connected to those past events. Therapists should allow ample opportunity for cancer survivors to talk about their pain and its meaning so that related past issues can be identified and addressed.

Appropriate use of medication, of course, is probably the most important way to reduce pain. According to Mullan and Hoffman (1990), 90 percent of people with cancer can have their pain effectively controlled through appropriate medication. However, cancer survivors sometimes do not know how to use medication for pain appropriately. They may believe they are being brave or strong by refusing medication as long as possible. In reality, according to LeShan (1989, p. 98), "Every study shows that people who receive their pain medication when the pain first starts need much less of it and ask for it less often than do people who wait until they can't stand it anymore." McGuire (1987) stressed the importance of a fixed schedule of medication in order to achieve optimal pain relief, reduce anxiety, improve quality of life, and reduce total amount of medication that is needed. Receiving medication as soon as needed for intermittent pain also can give cancer survivors a greater sense of control and can ease fears that they will have to cope with high levels of pain.

Another erroneous belief that may lead people to refuse needed medication is the fear of addiction. According to Breitbart and Passik (1993, p. 57), "Although tolerance and physical dependence commonly occur" with use of narcotic analgesics, "addiction (psychological dependence) is rare and almost never occurs in individuals without a history of drug abuse."

Therapists also should consider the possibility that secondary gains, perhaps attention and sympathy, are contributing to a person's experience of the pain. By involving close friends and family members in efforts to reduce the pain and by encouraging them to reinforce wellness behaviors rather than increased pain, therapists may be able to reduce the contribution of secondary gains (Golden, Gersh, & Robbins, 1992). However, this approach should be viewed as a last resort and used with great caution because it may be seen as manipulating the client.

Overview of Chapter

Psychotherapy can help cancer survivors in many ways. Not only can it modify distress, depression, anxiety, fear, and other negative emotional responses to the disease, it also can help people accept and cope effectively with their medical treatments, reducing pain, nausea, sexual dysfunction, and the impact on self-image of the aversive consequences of cancer and its treatments.

8

• •

Therapy and Support Groups

Many researchers have lent support to the use of group therapy with cancer survivors and have elaborated on the type of group therapy that is desirable. Bloom, Kang, and Romano (1991, p. 113) summarized the conclusions of those studies: "Results of several studies indicate that these interventions [group therapy] are perceived as enjoyable, increase knowledge about cancer and its treatment, reduce the severity of cancer symptoms such as pain, reduce dysphoria, improve self-esteem and sense of efficacy and may even lengthen survival in cancer patients."

Spiegel's research has been particularly important in demonstrating the value of group therapy for cancer survivors.

Spiegel's Research

David Spiegel, skeptical of the positive reports that were emerging of the beneficial effects of psychological interventions for people with cancer, developed a carefully designed study that he believed would dispel the belief that psychotherapy could make a difference. Spiegel and his colleagues (Spiegel, Bloom, & Yalom, 1981) studied two groups of women with metastatic breast cancer and a poor prognosis. The women were randomly divided between control and intervention groups. Women in the control group received only routine oncological care. Women in the intervention condition met weekly in groups of seven to ten members for ninety-minute sessions of supportive/expressive therapy. Interventions included such techniques as hypnosis to promote relaxation and alter the experience of pain, skill development (assertiveness, coping skills), and the opportunity to express feelings and receive support. The women were helped to take charge of their lives, become actively involved in their medical care, face their fears of dying, and reduce depression and pain.

After twelve months, differences in mood level, coping skills, pain, and energy level were found between the control group and the intervention group, with the intervention group showing considerable improvement in all these areas. The group therapy also seemed to have a significant impact on the women's health. Those in the control condition lived an average of 18.9 months after joining the study while those in the intervention group lived an average of 36.6 months after joining the study. Ten years after the beginning of the study, three women in the experimental group were still alive while all those in the control condition had died.

In explaining why group therapy had such a powerful impact, Spiegel (1992, pp. 115-116) wrote, "Cancer patients live with constant terror, yet have difficulty expressing their fears." Others do not receive their feelings easily, leading the cancer patients to withdraw and feel isolated, "as if they are already dead." When they can openly discuss their fears in a nonjudgmental context, they become "detoxified." Through supportive/expressive group therapy, the women gained a greater sense of control, became aware and tolerant of their strong feelings, and became better able to use social support. Reductions in pain as well as increased energy enabled them to become more active. Their moods as well as their quality of life improved.

Spiegel (1992, p. 117) found the differences in longevity "coherent with epidemiological evidence that the extent of a social network is associated with age-adjusted mortality." According to Spiegel, "Numerous studies suggest that suppression of negative affect, excessive conformity, severe stress, and lack of social support predict a poorer medical outcome with cancer. . . . Good psychosocial support may block this suppression. . . . Social support, especially support that enhances a patient's sense of control and assertiveness, seems to improve outcome" (pp. 118-119). He also suggested that the group therapy may have changed attitudes, leading to greater compliance with physician's recommendations on medication and diet, and thereby contributing to improved health.

In summarizing the essential ingredients of group therapy for cancer survivors, Spiegel (1992, p. 113) wrote, "Psychotherapeutic methods that have proved to be effective involve direct confrontation of fears; expression of affect, including negative feelings; provision of social support; and training in self-hypnosis for analgesia." He also observed that the effect of social support was likely to be most powerful for people in the early stages of cancer and that support from women was most strongly associated with health benefits for both men and women.

Other Studies

In addition to the approaches recommended by Spiegel, other interventions have also been found useful in group therapy for cancer survivors. Mathieson and Stam (1991) successfully used goal setting, behavioral rehearsal and role playing, self-monitoring, feedback and coaching, and homework between sessions to promote improvement in mood, coping skills, and adjustment. Hopwood and Maguire (1992) found that focusing on specific techniques that cancer survivors could learn and use to help themselves, such as relaxation, meditation, or imagery, was essential to the success of group therapy in reducing emotional distress and enhancing coping skills.

Fawzy et al. (1993) conducted an experimental study of the impact of structured group therapy on people with malignant melanoma. These groups consisted of seven to ten members and met for one and one-half hours weekly for six weeks, beginning an average of 112 days postsurgery. The group therapy had four components: (1) education on cancer and its treatments, (2) stress management, (3) enhancement of coping skills and problem solving, and (4) psychological support. In follow-up studies, members of the experimental group exhibited higher energy, greater use of active-behavioral coping, less depression and fatigue, and higher self-esteem than members of the control group (Fawzy et al., 1990). In addition, members of the experimental group had lower rates of recurrence and death at follow-up than did those in the control group. Fawzy et al. explained these findings by suggesting that the group experience fostered better health habits (such as nutrition, sun protection), effective coping, improved attitudes, treatment compliance, better physician-patient relationships, stress reduction, and social support and also may have improved immune system functioning.

Group therapy seems to reduce negative emotional reactions to radiation treatment. Decker, Cline-Elsen, and Gallagher (1992) compared people undergoing radiotherapy who also received six one-hour sessions of group therapy, including instruction in relaxation and opportunity to discuss concerns, to people who did not receive this intervention along with their radiation therapy. People in the experimental group demonstrated less tension, anger, fatigue, and depression than did people in the control group.

For women with early-stage cancer who are undergoing adjuvant medical treatment, Haber (1993) recommended a time-limited, structured group, perhaps only a single session of three hours' duration. She found that such a group could provide both support and skills without adding to the burden already experienced by women undergoing time-consuming medical procedures.

Telch and Telch (1986) studied cancer survivors who manifested clear evidence of psychological distress in an experiment that involved three conditions. People in the *coping group* received instruction in relaxation, stress management, cognitive restructuring, assertiveness, and goal setting. Homework assignments and role play were used. Those in the *support group* had the opportunity to discuss their feelings and concerns in an unstructured forum. Both groups met for six weekly sessions of ninety minutes. People in a *control condition* did not participate in group therapy. At the end of the treatment, the emotional distress of the people in the control condition had worsened. People in the support group showed reductions in anxiety and depression while those in the coping group improved not only on those measures but also in their activity level, their satisfaction with themselves, their communication skills, their ability to cope with medical procedures, and their sense of control and mastery. Based on these results, the authors concluded, "These results support providing psychologically distressed cancer patients with multifaceted coping skills training" (p. 802), and they support the use of the group context to teach those skills.

Similar results were obtained in a study by Cunningham and Tocco (1989). They too compared supportive group therapy with coping skills training. The supportive group included ventilation of feelings, information sharing, and discussion of problems associated with the diagnosis and treatment of cancer. The coping skills training taught progressive muscle relaxation, mental imagery and self-hypnosis, and also focused on lifestyle management, goal setting, and spiritual issues. Practice of new skills was encouraged both in the group and at home, with the aid of a workbook and audiotapes. While both groups were beneficial, the coping skills group had a more powerful impact.

Guidelines

Zimpfer (1989) summarized the goals of groups for cancer survivors as follows:

- Providing support
- Offering a place where emotions, no matter how strong or negative or unacceptable in other settings, can be shared

- Developing coping skills

- Receiving information and education

- Dealing with existential concerns, issues of guilt and mortality, as well as fears, hopes, and plans for the future

Haber (1993) and her colleagues, focusing on women with breast cancer, concluded that a supportive/expressive group could provide an opportunity for catharsis and unburdening, learning from role models and the knowledge and experience of others, and a feeling of hope and optimism. Group therapy can also promote self-esteem and relationship skills through the process of mutual helping. Guilt and self-blame can be reduced through learning that others have similar feelings and gaining perspective and objectivity on those feelings. Sharing successes and supporting each other through disappointments can build hope and enable participants to develop a vision of the future (Brigham, 1994). The rapid development of rapport and bonding that is common among cancer survivors reduces feelings of loneliness and alienation. Topics such as fear of death and recurrence, sexual problems, and self-blame, which may not be discussed anywhere else, can be shared in the group with acceptance and understanding.

Vugia (1991) reviewed the literature published between 1973 and 1989 on oncology support groups. The key elements of such groups were caring, esteem, and sharing. Most groups helped survivors and their families to maintain a social identity and receive emotional and environmental support, information, and social affiliation. The groups served as a stress buffer and helped people to cope and adapt to the diagnosis of cancer. Most groups were small (approximately seven members), closed, homogeneous groups conducive to the development of cohesiveness. Same-gender groups seemed especially helpful for discussion of sexual and other intimate issues.

Common themes in groups for cancer survivors included the following:

Intrapsychic: Anger, fear of death and pain, loneliness, denial, depression, guilt, hope, helplessness, the meaning of cancer, spiritual issues, memories, living for today

Interpersonal: Relationships, sexuality, dependence, loneliness, how much/whom to tell, disease progression, dealing with children and families, making wills

Social: Isolation, stigma, role and lifestyle changes

Cancer-related themes: Pain, side effects of treatment, treatment compliance, suicide, communication with medical staff, nontraditional treatments, finances, relapse

Brief, structured group meetings can accommodate considerable heterogeneity in membership. However, therapists should screen prospective members to ensure suitability. People who are extremely needy, angry, or withdrawn probably should receive some individual therapy before being placed in group therapy. In addition, isolates should be avoided; one person with advanced cancer should not be placed in a group in which all the other members have an excellent prognosis (Haber, 1993).

For People with Advanced Cancer

People with metastatic cancer typically need long-term group therapy, providing not only support and skill development but also help with depression and anxiety, fear of dying, pain control, family issues, and other concerns such as determining meaning and values in their lives, completing unfinished business, and developing the ability to meet the demands of dying (Selfridge, 1990). The shared common experience, the process of helping others, and the cohesiveness of the group can instill hope in participants that they can cope with the problems of dying and can give a sense of meaning to the time they have left. Homogeneity should be maximized in these groups to promote cohesiveness and sharing.

Special attention needs to be paid to resistance in these groups; the dying members may withdraw to avoid burdening others while the healthier members may withdraw out of fear of dealing with the deaths of other members. Sharing feelings and grieving together can counteract that withdrawal.

Special Challenges

Therapy groups for cancer survivors may have not only those difficulties common to most groups such as silences and problematic members but also may have difficulties related to the disease. Haber (1993) identified some common problems in therapy groups for cancer survivors. Resistance to the group experience may stem from shame about self-revelation; anxiety about being a burden to others in the group; apprehension related to hearing about the medical problems of others, especially recurrences and deaths; and lack of confidence that others can understand and be helpful. In addition, absences due to illness or medical treatment and competition to be the healthiest or sickest member of the group can be disruptive. Baron (1985) found that resistance in therapy groups for cancer survivors commonly took the form of dwelling on the distress associated with cancer or complaining about the medical establishment rather than seeking constructive solutions. Therapists need to set broad goals and use interventions that will enable group members to move past their disappointments. Defenses should be respected, but therapists can feel free to disagree and express their own perceptions.

Role of the Therapist

Vugia (1991) recommended that groups for cancer survivors have two leaders, one with medical training and one with psychological training. Ideally, one also should be a cancer survivor. Roles of the group leaders identified by Vugia included promoting cohesion, developing a safe climate, helping support to evolve, providing ample reinforcement, reducing stress, and giving information.

Groups for cancer survivors seem most helpful when the therapist initially is active, directive, and structured and then gradually allows the members to assume more control as they become comfortable and committed to the group process. Focus should be personal and practical, emphasizing emotions as well as cognitive-behavioral coping skills. Abstract discussions and intellectualization should be minimized. Eliciting common experiences can promote cohesiveness. Ensuring that members are acknowledged and responded to when they speak can also contribute to cohesiveness as well as to self-esteem and empowerment. Tapping into the anger of passive and depressed members can help to mobilize and energize them as well as involve them more fully in the group.

Model for Group Therapy

The following outline provides an overview of eight ninety-minute sessions of group therapy for cancer survivors. The worksheets included in Part B of the Resources section of this book are integrated into the sessions.

Session 1: The first session includes getting acquainted, setting the ground rules and goals for the group, initiating an atmosphere of acceptance and support, telling the members' stories, and presenting a task for completion between sessions (see Worksheet 1, "Writing About My Diagnosis," in Resource B).

Session 2: This session and all subsequent sessions begin with an opportunity for group members to talk about reactions or experiences they have had since the previous session. Focus of this session is on the relationship between cancer and emotions, with discussion centering on initial reactions to cancer and its treatments. Information, designed primarily to normalize reactions and reduce anxiety, is provided. Worksheet 2, "Ways to Help Myself Cope with Cancer," is the task for the next session.

Session 3: Initial discussion reviews participants' reactions to the worksheet they completed between sessions. Information is then provided on the importance of coping mechanisms. Behavioral techniques such as progressive muscle relaxation and focused breathing that can reduce stress are demonstrated. Tasks for completion after the session include implementation of behavioral coping mechanisms.

Session 4: Cognitive and cognitive-behavioral interventions are the focus of this session, with particular attention paid to teaching group members to identify and dispute cognitive distortions. A visualization exercise is used with the group, in which participants imagine their inner guide and begin to use the guide as a source of information and support. Tasks between sessions include practicing visualization.

Session 5: This session deals with participants' relationships outside the group and how they have been affected by cancer. Techniques are presented to improve assertiveness and communication skills and strengthen natural support systems. Worksheet 3, "Facilitating Difficult Conversations About Cancer," is completed for session 6.

Session 6: After discussion of Worksheet 3 and of efforts to improve relationships, focus shifts to a presentation of additional information on the relationship between cancer and emotions. Using Worksheet 4, "Qualities and Life Circumstances that May Be Associated with Prognosis," participants generate ways they can maximize those qualities associated with a positive prognosis. Individual tasks are planned to increase hardiness and a fighting spirit.

Session 7: This session focuses on identifying and coping with continuing fears, using Worksheet 5, "Coping with the Fear of Recurrence or Treatment Failure." Participants are encouraged to identify their current cancer-related fears and explore ways they might deal with them successfully. Individual tasks are drawn from Worksheet 5 for completion between sessions.

Session 8: If this is the final group session, it will include some time for processing the group experience and reinforcement of positive changes participants have made. Future goals will be established to improve emotional and physical health. Worksheet 6, "Goal Setting," is used to facilitate that process.

Additional sessions might include guest speakers (such as oncologists, surgeons, long-term cancer survivors). In addition, each session may be extended to afford a longer group experience. This model can be adapted to provide a structure for short-term group therapy with almost any cancer survivors.

The Cancer Survivor as Group Member

Only 10 to 29 percent of cancer survivors participate in self-help or psychotherapy groups (Hopwood & Maguire, 1992). Mathieson and Stam (1991) studied cancer survivors who sought out support groups and found they did not seem more troubled than survivors who did not initiate involvement in such groups. Several variables did distinguish the two groups. People who joined support groups were more aware of their concerns, were more likely to be white females, and were more likely to have had negative experiences with the medical community. Another study (Bauman, Gervey, & Siegel, 1992) found that people most likely to participate in support groups were well-educated, under age fifty, unmarried, members of other voluntary organizations, and in contact with mental health professionals. People with a Protestant religious affiliation were more likely to use support groups than people from Catholic or Jewish backgrounds. Extent of social support did not determine whether people sought out support groups; people with little social support as well as those with considerable social support participated in support groups specifically for cancer survivors. Most often expressed reasons for attending support groups included the wish to compare one's emotional and physical progress with others, to learn more about the disease, and to share concerns with others who would understand.

Group Versus Individual Therapy

Baron (1985) asserted that group therapy had many advantages over one-to-one therapy for cancer survivors. The group provides a safe place in which to share fears and feelings with others and can pave the way for better communication in the outside world. Group members can provide a credible source of reality testing on the disease and can confront one another's denial without creating barriers between therapist and client. The group can exert pressure on a negative or self-destructive member in a way that the therapist cannot; members of one group made a group telephone call to a member who had dropped out of a group and then appeared at her home before the next group meeting to escort her to group. Farash (1979) found that self-help groups were as effective as individual psychotherapy in helping women resolve concerns around body image following mastectomies. While some cancer survivors prefer and probably would benefit more from individual therapy, the group setting seems especially appropriate for addressing the concerns of cancer survivors.

Natural Support Systems

Natural support systems also can contribute to both the emotional and physical well-being of cancer survivors. Friends, family, neighbors, and colleagues can all provide support and understanding as well as practical help such as child care, meal preparation, information gathering, and rides to medical treatments.

Some evidence is available that social support is related to mortality. Bloom, Kang, and Romano (1991) found that people who were married had lower mortality rates than did those who were single, widowed, or divorced. They also found that people with more social interactions and larger social networks had lower mortality rates than those who were isolated. They offered three possible explanations for the connection between social support and mortality: (1) the direct effect of social support on stress, (2) a buffering effect, in which social support reduces the impact of stress, and (3) an effect on health unrelated to stress in which people who have the skills to develop social supports as well as the encouragement and motivation provided by their support systems take better care of themselves and have better coping skills. For example, breast self-examination is more likely to be practiced by women who have friends and family members who also practice breast self-examination. Social support may also promote earlier medical attention and treatment of disease as well as better adherence to difficult medical regimens.

Women are more successful at obtaining support than men. Jevne (1990) found that 64 percent of women in an oncology treatment facility in Alberta, Canada, were receiving moderate to strong support, while 58 percent of the men received only weak support. Whether this is due to the greater involvement with friends and family that women seem to have, the women's greater ability to express their needs and ask for help, or the perception of others that the men needed less help is unclear. However, therapists may need to give men additional help in developing their support systems. Low levels of support were also more common among people with multiple problems, strong anger and depression, marital and parenting difficulties, and financial concerns. Ways to help people develop and make good use of their natural support systems will be discussed further in the next chapter.

Structured Peer Support Groups

In addition to professionally led support groups discussed earlier in this chapter, groups led by paraprofessionals or other cancer survivors are also available. The American Cancer Society, for example, offers short-term groups led by long-term cancer survivors in which approximately ten people, newly diagnosed with the same type of cancer, have an opportunity to meet. These groups provide support, reduce isolation, and allow opportunity to discuss intimate personal concerns, such as the impact of cancer on sexuality and religious beliefs, with others who are likely to have similar concerns. Although groups such as these focus primarily on the newly diagnosed, groups may be encouraged to continue meeting independently after the planned sessions. My own support group has continued to meet monthly for more than five years.

Even for people with ample support systems, structured support groups can help people better utilize their natural support systems and can make some contributions that perhaps can only be made by other cancer survivors, such as reducing isolation and stigma and providing role models and firsthand information on successfully coping with cancer and its treatments. According to Spiegel (Moyers, 1993, p. 68), "The act of merely being with and interacting with others who face a similar experience serves to buffer the traumatic effects of facing an illness on one's own."

Types of Support

Many varieties of support are available to cancer survivors. In the Reach to Recovery program, sponsored by the American Cancer Society, women hospitalized because of surgery for breast cancer are visited by long-term survivors who had similar surgery. The visitors provide support, information, a temporary prosthesis, and an encouraging role model. One forty-six-year-old woman who had extensive lymph node involvement, a negative prognostic sign, was visited by a sixty-six-year-old survivor who had the same lymph node involvement when she was diagnosed with breast cancer twenty years earlier. Seeing that it was possible to survive her disease gave the patient the sort of hope that the physicians had not been able to provide her.

Another short-term intervention, providing information and peer support, is the Look Good, Feel Better program. Volunteers with expertise in makeup and hair styles meet with groups of cancer survivors to provide information on dealing with the impact of cancer and its treatment on the appearance. Participants are given samples of cosmetics and taught to conceal such cancer-related changes as pallor, loss of eyebrows and eyelashes, and discolorations. Sample wigs, hairpieces, and turbans are displayed and tried on. The camaraderie provided by a group of balding, fatigued women experimenting with new hairstyles and makeup is somehow uplifting. Manne, Girasek, and Ambrosino (1994) found that the Look Good, Feel Better program significantly improved mood and feelings of attractiveness, reduced anxiety, normalized changes, provided welcome support and attention, and distracted the participants from their worries.

Drop-In Support Groups

Another model for peer support groups is drop-in groups that are offered by hospitals and other treatment facilities for people with cancer. These programs typically are open to cancer survivors as well as their family members and include people with many types of cancer in various stages of the disease. Such groups are readily accessible in most communities and can offer support and information.

Because of the diversity of the membership in these groups, time spent on the details of any one person's medical condition may be curtailed as may be comparisons of symptoms and prognoses. Membership in such groups usually is not controlled or predetermined. As a result, a group meeting may be too large or too small to provide a comfortable arena for self-expression and support. Because these groups usually are heterogeneous, people with varied prognoses may meet together. This may lead people with good prognoses to become more fearful after interaction with people with advanced disease while those with poor prognoses may not receive the time and attention they need. Heterogeneous groups such as these are helpful to some cancer survivors but should be recommended with care.

For Children and Families

Many types of groups are available for cancer survivors and their families. Some groups combine cancer survivors and family members, some are only for survivors, while others are restricted to family members or partners of those with cancer. Family and friends of cancer survivors often benefit more from having their own group. That enables them to express themselves more freely, without fear of upsetting the survivor. Even their most disturbing feelings such as wishes for the death of a loved one with advanced cancer or loss of sexual desire for a partner who has undergone extensive surgery can be expressed, understood, accepted, and normalized in a family support group.

Adolescents in particular seem to benefit from groups comprised solely of teenagers whose parents or siblings have cancer. Such groups seem to allow them to express concerns and feelings that they are reluctant to disclose to their family members or to other adults.

Therapists should familiarize themselves with the support groups available in their communities and assist cancer survivors and their families to locate the most appropriate support groups. The following are some types of groups that have helped people cope with cancer.

Knakal (1988) described a couples group with a maximum of sixteen members in which one member of each couple had cancer. The goals of the group were to enable the couples to regain their previous levels of functioning by sharing experiences and coping strategies with others and receiving support and information. Major themes included anger at the cancer survivor for getting sick, fear of abandonment, and difficulty coping with role changes.

Another vehicle for providing support is a specialized camp. These camps are increasing in number, with most designed to provide social support as well as information and skill development to children with cancer.

Parent advocate programs are yet another relatively new form of support. Such a program has been set up at the University of Rochester Medical Center. In that program, parents who have dealt with their children's cancer treatments are available to provide empathy, support, information, and role models to parents whose children have recently been diagnosed with cancer. According to the authors (Carpenter et al., 1992, p. 27), "The provision of peer support by individuals who have had personal experience with a particular crisis can be a vital component in facilitating the adjustment of others who are confronted with the same crisis." Carpenter et al. also found however that careful selection of the parent advocates was important in determining their effectiveness and that the advocates needed their own support group to help them deal with the challenges and stress of helping others cope with cancer.

School-based groups for children who have family members with cancer are a resource that seems to be increasing in availability. Call (1990) found that the process of sharing and being listened to was most important to the participants of such groups. Children benefited from having a specific time to express their feelings. School-based support groups also helped children reduce their isolation, receive reassurance and support, obtain clear information, feel involved and important, normalize their reactions, reduce the stigma they were experiencing, and plan ways to maintain age-appropriate interests and activities. Call found that groups could combine children whose parents were cancer survivors with those with other family members who had cancer, as long as no one child had a very different experience from the others. However, Call recommended separate groups for children coping with bereavement.

Sourkes (1991) made effective use of art therapy with pediatric oncology patients as well as with their siblings. The children were asked to create several drawings: a color-feeling wheel to represent their emotions, a drawing of the changes in their families, and a drawing of their fears. Discussion, as well as the process of drawing, helped to reduce upset and normalize feelings. Letter writing, as well as drawings, were used to help children whose siblings already had died. Techniques such as these may be helpful to adults as well as to children.

Another approach to helping children with a family member who has cancer was a curriculum for health professionals to use with these children. Sullivan (1990), for example, described a wealth of useful and creative activities, lessons, and exercises that could be used to help children deal with the impact of cancer on their families. Representative activities included the following:

- "Cancer Explorers" (taught children about the causes of cancer)

- Gibberish exercise (focused attention on how cancer disrupts family communication)

- Group fantasy

- Journals (for artistic expression, recording of feelings and ideas)

- Dictionary (developed by each participant, explained terms and concepts associated with cancer)

- Role plays of conversations with family members

- Sentence completions (a vehicle for identifying and exploring feelings)

- Psychodramas (to explore roles and important incidents in the families)

- Writing a story about one's family, before and after cancer

- Hospital tours

- Using puppets to express feelings

- Group brainstorming (to generate ways to solve problems)

Support groups for adolescents and young adults coping with cancer are especially necessary because of the importance of peer support and issues of identity in those age groups. Ettinger and Heiney (1993) described a program called Lasting Impressions that used support groups to help young people and their families cope with the diagnosis and treatment of cancer, to promote community reentry, and to enhance their long-term readjustment. The groups were designed to give support, normalize concerns, promote mastery of developmental tasks, improve coping skills, increase understanding of the disease, build self-esteem by developing a sense of responsibility and pride in one's accomplishments, improve social skills, and build relationships with peers and families. Monthly support groups as well as three retreats per year were held for the survivors. Parents had their own support groups as well as three "nights out" a year. The participants wrote and produced a monthly newsletter and a membership directory, offered peer visitation, and had a broad range of creative and service activities designed to promote contact, cohesiveness, and a sense of accomplishment.

Benefits and Drawbacks

What seems most important in determining the impact of support is a person's perception of that support rather than the actual nature and amount of the support. Stam, Koopmans, and Mathieson (1991), studying the impact of support on people whose cancer treatment involved laryngectomies, found that perceived, rather than received, support had a stress-buffering impact and promoted improvement in mood and recovery of functioning.

The following quotations from interviews with cancer survivors capture many of the benefits provided by support groups:

"My emotional well-being comes in large part from my interaction with other women with breast cancer. . . . There is an instant bonding. I discovered that anger, denial, suicidal thoughts, depression, anxiety, and fear of recurrence are common reactions. No feeling is too crazy or too awful to be accepted by these women."

"You are helped as you help. Real recovery begins when you help someone else experiencing all the feelings and fears you did."

"Support groups help me feel less isolated, less guilty, more informed; they've made me more politically active."

Not all reactions to support groups are positive. This is evident in quotations such as "One support group I went to was depressing because everybody there was depressed" and "I identify with anyone who has cancer. Their disappointments and deaths become very personalized and too painful for me." Cancer survivors who are in extreme denial, who are very fragile, or who are experiencing serious mental disorders probably would benefit more from individual therapy than from a peer support group or even a psychotherapy group. Perhaps once they have made progress through individual therapy, they will be able to benefit from a support group but this should be carefully integrated into their overall treatment.

Greer (van Rood & Balner, 1990) found that given the choice, most cancer survivors preferred individual therapy to group therapy. However, little comparative research has been conducted to determine the effectiveness of each approach in helping cancer survivors. Group therapy may sound more intimidating, particularly to people without prior experience in psychotherapy. However, for people who are not experiencing severe mental disorders, group therapy actually may be more beneficial. Therapists should be sure that people understand the potential benefits and drawbacks that peer support or therapy groups can offer and weigh both clients' preferences and their apparent needs before making treatment recommendations. However, exposure to other cancer survivors who are not faring well medically should not necessarily be viewed as harmful to those people with good prognoses.

Even people who are functioning reasonably well and who can benefit from a peer support group will feel sorrow or anxiety in response to other members' experiences. In less than a year, two members of a cancer support group with which I was consulting died. The deaths of course heightened the fears of the remaining members and evoked strong feelings of grief and anger. At the same time, the group members felt gratified that they had stood by the two members who died, visiting them in the hospital even when one was unable to speak because of a brain tumor, and planned ways to celebrate and remember the contributions of the two members after their deaths. This process helped the surviving members to cope with their grief and fears effectively and reassured them that if they too had a recurrence of their disease, they would have the full support of the group and would not be forgotten.

Groups have a great deal to offer to cancer survivors. Peer support groups, as well as professionally led therapy groups for cancer survivors, can provide the following benefits:

- Normalizing strong reactions to the diagnosis of cancer

- Enhancing feelings of self-worth and self-esteem through helping others and receiving reinforcement

- Creating a sense of belonging, reducing isolation

- Providing information that demystifies shared experiences and gives direction to coping

- Providing help with specific common problems (for example, sharing ways to overcome anticipatory nausea, driving someone to a medical appointment)

- Reducing emotional distress through ventilation and empathy

- Increasing self-efficacy and coping skills through modeling and suggestions

- Mobilizing the cancer survivor and giving direction to actions

- Reducing fear of the process of dying

- Encouraging health-enhancing behaviors

Overview of Chapter

Membership in groups, whether they are natural support groups, peer support groups, or professionally led psychotherapy groups, alone or in combination with individual or family therapy, can make a great difference in the emotional and physical health of people who are coping with cancer. Therapists should suggest these groups to their clients, help them address any reservations they might have about participating in support groups, and teach them to contribute to and benefit from their groups.

9

• •

Relationships and Cancer

Cancer, like any serious illness, affects not only the person with the disease but also family, friends, neighbors, co-workers, and others who have an important relationship with the cancer survivor. This chapter discusses the likely impact of cancer on the partners, children, parents, siblings, friends, and colleagues of a person with the disease and will present ways to help survivors and the important people in their lives have rewarding relationships in the face of cancer.

A reciprocal relationship has also been noted: cancer both affects relationships and is affected by relationships. People with cancer whose relationships are difficult or unrewarding may have a poorer medical outcome. Sabbioni (1991), for example, reported that women with a poor marriage, women who had recently been separated, and family caretakers of people with Alzheimer's disease had signs of a weaker immune system than people without those family difficulties. People with few social ties or activities have been found to have a particularly high death rate during the nine-year period surveyed by one study (Berkman & Syme, 1979). On the other hand, positive immune system activity has been associated with the perception of high-quality emotional support from one's spouse or partner as well as perceived social support from one's physician and use of social support as a coping strategy (Sabbioni, 1991). According to Zimpfer (1992, p. 208), "The likelihood of recovery is enhanced if one has strong support from whoever is seen as important (e.g., spouse, parent, child, employer, friend, neighbor, clergy person)."

Providing Support to the Cancer Survivor

Cancer survivors typically want and benefit from having a great deal of support. Emotional support, as well as the opportunity to communicate with significant others about fears and reactions to the diagnosis of cancer, has been found to reduce anxiety, guilt, hostility, and depression and to promote adjustment in cancer survivors (Gotcher, 1992). However, not all efforts to help are successful. The following quotations reflect cancer survivors' views of the kind of support that was helpful to them as well as their recollections of interactions that were hurtful to them.

What Cancer Survivors Found Helpful

"It has been a wonderfully uplifting and positive year emotionally. I have been wrapped in a warm blanket of love and support from family and friends."

"The most helpful responses have been the ones when I know the person is genuinely trying to listen and understand what living with cancer is like."

"I sought out anyone who would listen nonjudgmentally; most people acted as though they knew why I had cancer or were ready to tell me everything was all right. It was a rare individual who was willing to listen without offering a quick fix."

"Saying the right thing is pretty near impossible . . . but listening and asking the right questions was more valuable to me. . . . Just having people ask how I was let me know that they cared."

"Someone told me, 'You won't always feel this bad.' I have carried that thought with me."

"I liked it when people said they admired me. It says you're managing."

"It is reassuring when you are told that someone is with you and will help you no matter what it takes, no matter how long, no matter the effort, no conditions."

"Helpful responses were nonjudgmental, positive, and honest. Many people just let me talk and that was very helpful."

What Cancer Survivors Found Hurtful

"It was hurtful when people said, 'Let me tell you something worse' or 'Life goes on; stop talking about cancer,' or when they minimize what you have gone through."

"I tried to talk with my husband and sister about dying. They didn't want to hear it. They both said I had a good prognosis and so why worry about it?"

"I asked my family to read just one book on cancer. None of them have done so. This has saddened me."

"One member of my family ignored the positive and expanded upon the down times. That was difficult."

"Least helpful was when people said, 'You'll be fine' or 'It's all for the best' or telling you what to do. You can't tell another person what's going to be helpful to them."

"The worst was when people said, 'It's God's will' or 'God never gives you more than you can handle.'"

"Hurtful responses were ones that attempted a quick fix and laid a guilt trip on me. 'Negative thinking causes cancer, people with cancer don't eat properly, haven't you been taking care of yourself? did the doctor tell you to lose weight? is this something that should have been detected earlier?' were all lines I heard."

Guidelines for Providing Support

Friends and family members of people with cancer often are uncertain how to help and what to say and may seek guidance from psychotherapists on how to communicate with their loved ones who have been diagnosed with cancer. Based on my work with cancer survivors, as well as structured interviews with survivors, I have found these approaches to be the most supportive:

- Give the survivors the opportunity to talk about whatever they want to talk about, even if it seems depressing or discouraging.

- Listen carefully to what is being said, and show survivors they are heard by demonstrating empathy and asking questions about what they are saying.

- Emphasize the positive and praise the courage and strength of the cancer survivor in a truthful way, but do not minimize or disregard the negative.

- Avoid telling people what they did wrong or what they should do differently; be nonjudgmental.

- Avoid telling stories about other people with cancer, especially if the outcome is negative.

- Rather than offering specific advice or help to cancer survivors, ask what would be helpful to them and then try to meet their needs.

- Give messages of support that encourage rather than pressure; statements such as "I can't survive without you" can increase the survivor's anxiety and fear.

- Don't try to solve the problem or make things all right; that is impossible. All that is needed is to communicate caring, interest, involvement, and commitment to being there for the survivor.

Types of Support

Dakof and Taylor (1990) interviewed people with cancer to determine what they found to be helpful or unhelpful from potential support providers. They identified the following three types of helpful support:

1. *Esteem/emotional support:* Being present; expressing concern, empathy, or affection; communicating acceptance; expressing understanding; being kind and pleasant

2. *Informational support:* Providing information, serving as a positive role model, being optimistic about the person's prognosis and ability to cope with the disease

3. *Tangible support:* Providing practical help as needed and requested; providing competent medical care

The type of help most important to cancer survivors varies depending on the survivor's relationship with the person providing the support. From their spouses, people most valued their physical presence, concern and affection, and calm acceptance of the diagnosis. They were troubled by spouses who criticized how they were responding to the disease or minimized the impact of the disease. Concern and affection were the most important forms of support from other family members, while criticism and minimization again were most upsetting. Friends and acquaintances who offered concern and affection, practical assistance, and calm acceptance were appreciated while those who avoided contact, were pessimistic, intrusive, or inappropriate were not viewed positively. Other cancer survivors were valued for providing a special kind of understanding, information about cancer and its treatment, and role models, particularly if they demonstrated optimism, strength, and determination to enjoy the present. Finally, medical personnel were prized for offering accurate information, practical help, competent care, optimism, and concern and for being pleasant and kind. Dakof and Taylor's study supports my own findings that emotional support, especially acceptance, concern, affection, and optimism, generally is the most important type of support for cancer survivors.

The Impact of Cancer on Family Dynamics

For most cancer survivors, their families will be their primary source of support. The diagnosis of cancer can affect families in many ways. It can raise fears of loss and change. It can drain emotional and financial resources. It can deprive healthy family members of the support and attention they are used to because of the special needs of the cancer survivor. It can change roles, causing some family members to take on unfamiliar and unwanted tasks that at least temporarily can no longer be performed by the cancer survivor. Finally, it can cause enduring changes in the family's goals and lifestyle; fertility, parenting, sexuality, employability, as well as other important areas of functioning may be altered or impaired. At least 25 percent of families have significant emotional difficulties in response to a diagnosis of cancer (Sales, Schultz, & Biegel, 1992). (Readers interested in understanding the impact of cancer on families are referred to Chapter Two for information on assessing the family context.)

The extent of the stress that cancer puts on the family seems to be determined by two sets of variables (Sales, Schultz, & Biegel, 1992):

1. *Objective factors of the disease:* Severity, suddenness, patient's level of distress, site of the cancer, prognosis, duration of disease, nature and consequences of its treatment, and the demands on the caregivers

2. *Family context variables:* Composition of the family, health, income, social supports, relationships, personality factors, coping strategies, age, developmental stage, presence of other stressors, and background variables

Particularly stressful for families are long illnesses with poor prognoses that place high demands on caregivers in a family context that already is under pressure or dysfunctional. On the other hand, families that are cohesive; have flexible roles and belief systems; have minimal conflict; and have clear, frequent and open communication are likely to deal with cancer successfully. In fact, coping with cancer as a family actually can strengthen relationships (Sales, Schultz, & Biegel, 1992). Better survival rates also are associated with these positive family dynamics.

Most families will mobilize themselves to cope with cancer, provide the help and support that is needed, and then return to normal (Haber, 1993). Families typically handle cancer as they have handled other family crises and stressors. Families that were strong and cohesive initially seem most successful at coping effectively with cancer and its treatment while maintaining some internal stability. However, other families may deteriorate in the face of cancer and fail to provide needed support to the survivor as well as to maintain the stability needed by other family members.

Harmful Family Responses to Cancer

Common ways to deal with cancer that usually are harmful or discouraging to both the cancer survivor and other family members include the following:

Forced cheerfulness. This stance can lead survivors to become more pessimistic in order to establish the legitimacy of their reactions. Holding in their true feelings also can lead to depression and anxiety in family members. As Doan and Gray (1992, p. 263) stated, "In some instances, the cancer patient's family members, believing that the maintenance of a sense of well-being is vital to survival, will not tolerate any expression of fear, apprehension, discouragement or doubt by the patient. Far from being supportive, these well-intentioned efforts to promote the heroic response frequently leave the cancer patient feeling alienated, rejected and misunderstood."

Rejection/blame of the survivor. In an effort to regain some sense of control and to manage their own fears, families may blame the survivor and manifest shame and repugnance at the survivor's physical changes.

Rescuing the survivor. Families may exaggerate the helplessness of cancer survivors in an effort to support them, stripping them of their usual roles and responsibilities. This overprotection is likely to damage the survivors' self-esteem and may make them feel hopeless and useless.

Guilt and self-doubts. Family members may criticize themselves and feel inadequate because they view themselves as unable to help the cancer survivor. Open communication with medical staff and the survivor may clarify what the family can realistically contribute and how important that is, as well as what is out of its control.

Anticipatory grief and separation. Family members may distance themselves from the cancer survivor, in expectation of the person's death. This pattern is especially likely in small or very cohesive families where the survivor has a critical role. Family members may be feeling guilt, loneliness, sadness, denial, resentment, exhaustion, or the wish to escape (Rolland, 1994). These reactions can lead the survivor to feel isolated and abandoned and have been associated with a poor medical outcome.

Expecting business as usual. In an effort to deny their fears or to prevent the survivor from focusing on cancer, some families act as though little has happened and try to maintain family life just as it was before the diagnosis. Adoption of rigid patterns to maintain homeostasis and denial of uncertainty also may reflect a fear that the disease will worsen in the face of change (McDaniel, Hepworth, & Doherty, 1992). While maintaining some stability and continuity is important, denial of the impact of the disease can be destructive to both survivors and family members who must suppress their real feelings.

Acting out and frenetic activity. Family members may try to avoid the emotional pain of dealing with cancer by losing themselves in activities. Of particular concern are self-destructive behaviors such as conduct problems in children and substance abuse.

Helping Families Cope with Cancer

Family counseling with all or part of a survivor's family, including the survivor, can reduce stress in the family, counteract harmful responses, and build healthy coping mechanisms (Doka, 1993). Rolland (1994) believed that all families dealing with serious illness should have a mental health consultation to build their coping skills and promote self-expression. Encouraging families to develop and use active listening skills, to express their feelings openly but with sensitivity, and to focus on the positive can prevent their falling into some of the negative patterns discussed above. As much as possible, life as it was before cancer should go on, with particular emphasis being paid to maintaining family rituals and rewarding activities. Rituals involving celebration and affirmation can coalesce the family; other rituals can help them deal with loss (Rolland, 1994).

Efforts to maintain family stability should take account of the needs of the cancer survivor. Most cancer survivors need a great deal of help and support. Unifying the family into a team that will work together can provide both practical and emotional support to the survivor. Therapists can best accomplish this if they respect the family's coping style, normalize their negative feelings, and strengthen their cohesiveness. Any dysfunctional or destructive behaviors such as a child's acting out or a spouse avoiding closeness with the cancer survivor should be dealt with gently and gradually, focusing on feelings and reactions rather than blame. Empathy and support on the part of the therapist are essential.

The family's request for psychotherapy should be viewed not as a shortcoming or failure but as an effort to get as much help as possible. Family members should be congratulated for their concern and efforts. Empowerment of the family is important; therapists may provide tools, ideas, and information, but family efficacy should be developed by encouraging family members to take control and responsibility and by reinforcing the family's strengths and sense of identity.

To maintain a sense of empowerment in families in the face of uncertainty, therapists should emphasize hope and optimism but also should be realistic. They need to help families acknowledge the possibility of loss and to build flexibility in family roles, plans, and coping skills (Rolland, 1994). "What if" questions can be useful, such as, "The prognosis sounds very positive for a full recovery, but what if there is a relapse? How do you think this family would handle that?" Family efficacy can also be promoted by helping families discuss and arrive at decisions together and by helping families deal more effectively with health care professionals.

Families usually create their own meanings and explanations for unfortunate events. Exploring the meanings the family has given to the diagnosis of cancer can shed light on their use of coping mechanisms. For example, the family that blames the survivor for the disease may withdraw and appear rejecting while the family who believes the disease has genetic origins may become overprotective of its children. Discussion of family background, especially religious beliefs and prior experiences with serious illness, can be helpful in promoting understanding of the family's reactions to the present disease.

Transitions are common for families dealing with life-threatening illness, including the transition from diagnosis to treatment, from treatment to recovery, and sometimes the transitions to relapse and death. These usually involve change, upheaval, and reevaluation. Although transitions are difficult, they also can be windows of opportunity for change, times when the family is particularly receptive to intervention (Rolland, 1994).

Caregivers and other family members need support too, as does the cancer survivor. Therapists can help other family members to express their needs for help and support and help the family function in a mutually supportive fashion.

Gathering Information from the Family

In psychotherapy with a family coping with cancer, the entire family or caregiving system should be involved, not just the survivor.

A comprehensive initial interview with a family affected by cancer might include exploration of the following areas:

- *Expectations for therapy.* Especially if the family is not self-referred, the session might begin with a brief discussion of how the family believes psychotherapy can be helpful to them, their understanding of therapy, and an explanation by the therapist of that process, emphasizing the importance of family cohesiveness and empowerment.
- *Identifying the family.* Who are the significant members of the family? This might include close friends or colleagues as well as relatives.
- *Family structure and dynamics.* What systems and subsystems operate in the family? What patterns of closeness and communication are evident? What are the usual roles and responsibilities in the family? Have these been determined by gender, age, preference, abilities, or other dimensions? Particular attention should be paid to the organization of the family, the distribution of influence and power, and the patterns and nature of communication (McDaniel, Hepworth, & Doherty, 1992).
- *Telling one's own story.* Just as the cancer survivor has a story, so does the family. Family members each should be given the opportunity to describe how they learned about the diagnosis, what their understanding of the disease is, and what their reactions have been. Enmeshed families may expect everyone to view the disease in the same way, while in other families, differences in beliefs or attitudes may be intensified by the crisis of the disease. Ideally, through these stories, the therapist can develop understanding not only of family perceptions of the disease and its cause but of the actual nature of the disease, its treatment, its physical consequences, and its prognosis.
- *Impact of cancer on the family.* Both the actual and the feared or anticipated impact of the disease should be explored, with particular attention being paid to changes in roles and family lifestyle,

affective and behavioral symptoms presented by family members (such as acting out, depression, changes in sleeping and eating), and practical concerns (finances, child care, management of the home).

• *Family context*. Information on developmental stages, values and religious beliefs, and concurrent family concerns can help put the diagnosis of cancer in context and yield a fuller understanding of family responses to the diagnosis. Typically, coping with a serious illness causes a family to solidify and pull inward (Rosen, 1990). If the family had been at a very different developmental stage prior to the diagnosis, in which boundaries were loosening, such as the stage of the adolescent children moving out of the home, conflict in the family may be heightened. Similarly, families in transition or coping with other serious concerns may have particular difficulty coping with yet another stressor. Concurrent difficulties may become confused with the problems associated with cancer or may even be blamed for the cancer; one cancer survivor blamed his cancer on the conflict he had been having with his wife.

Families with young children who are already coping with busy lives and multiple roles and demands usually have more difficulty adapting to a diagnosis of cancer than do older families who may have more stability and resources and may not be as surprised by the diagnosis. Families with rigid belief systems also tend to have particular difficulty in dealing with serious illness and may feel shame, failure, and loss of control at their inability to prevent or resolve difficulties related to the disease.

• *How the family has coped with other losses, crises, and problems*. This background information will shed light on the adequacy of the family's coping skills and typical coping style.

• *Previous family experience with serious illness*. A genogram, discussed in Chapter Two, can be useful in promoting exploration of family history, serious illnesses and causes of death, and family patterns of coping with illness. Current coping styles and ways of responding to illness are likely to reflect those of the past.

• *Family resources*. Financial, educational, spiritual, and interpersonal resources should be explored. Particularly important is identification of support systems and social networks, friends, family, neighbors, clergy, and colleagues who might be able to assist the family. Relationships with health professionals also should be discussed.

• *Progress and expectations*. How has the family dealt with the disease thus far? What problems have they encountered? What problems do they anticipate? How well has the family functioned as a team? Who seems to need special help? What do the family members see in the future? What are their strengths? What do they want their life after cancer to be like?

Assessment of the Family

A comprehensive interview, as well as observation of the family, should give therapists insight into the following important areas of family functioning:

- Family membership, hierarchy, systems, and subsystems

- Nature of family boundaries (rigid, flexible, or weak)

- How enmeshed or disengaged the family is

- Whether the family is underfunctioning, overfunctioning, or adequately functioning

- Styles of communication and patterns of interaction

- Developmental patterns and issues

- Unresolved issues that may impair the family's ability to cope with cancer

- Impact of family history, especially of illness and loss

- Experience with past and present stressors

- Response to cancer, including secondary gains associated with the disease such as special attention or power

- Family strengths and coping mechanisms

When a Partner Has Cancer

If the cancer survivor is married or in a committed relationship, the process of coping with the disease will inevitably affect the couple relationship. The partner typically will have intense, conflicting, seemingly irrational feelings, usually including anger as well as guilt and grief (Rolland, 1994). Barraclough (1994) reported that depression and anxiety are almost as common among partners as among cancer survivors: 50 percent of partners have some symptoms of depression and anxiety, with 25 percent experiencing severe symptoms. A survey of partners of women who had been diagnosed with breast cancer yielded the following important areas of concern, listed in descending order of frequency reported:

1. *Reacting to the illness:* Gathering information, making decisions, dealing with the health care system

2. *Negotiating the illness experience:* Shock, fear, loss, moodiness, eating and sleeping problems, fatigue

3. *Adapting lifestyle to meet the demands of the illness:* Changes in work schedule, child care, social changes, coping with the constant presence of the disease

4. *Being sensitive to the cancer survivor's needs:* Trying to be supportive and consoling, feeling leaned on, bearing the brunt of the survivor's anger and upset

5. *Thinking about the future:* Uncertainty, fears of recurrence and death, anxiety

6. *Attempting to minimize the effects of the illness:* Looking to the future, emphasizing the positive

7. *Feeling the impact of cancer on the relationship and on communication*

Issues for Cancer Survivors and Their Partners

Cancer survivors sometimes become demanding and angry toward their partners for not understanding or helping enough. As one cancer survivor put it, "I was filled with anger. . . . I was angry at having cancer and even angrier that my family didn't understand. They all had assumed I was strong and capable of handling anything. They saw a me they did not recognize." On the other hand, some cancer survivors withdraw from their partners and may even compromise their medical treatments to avoid becoming a burden or being rejected by their partners (Winograd, 1992).

The impact of the disease can serve as a catalyst to raise long-standing relationship problems that may be resolved in the course of dealing with cancer or may lead to a breakdown of the relationship. Haber (1993) reported that 7 percent of marriages end after a woman has been diagnosed with breast cancer, usually at the wife's initiation. Cancer survivors become more aware of their mortality and may no longer be willing to put up with unrewarding or destructive relationships. On the other hand, Hughes (1987) surveyed sixty-seven married couples in which one partner had cancer and found that sixty-one reported their marriages were the same or closer after dealing with cancer. Some relationships become enmeshed following cancer, perhaps in reaction to fears of losing the partner to cancer (Carter, Carter, & Siliunas, 1993).

The disease will probably cause a change in roles and responsibilities. This may be especially difficult for couples who have maintained well-differentiated roles, following traditional gender expectations. As one survivor said, "Even though I frequently was too sick to eat, the responsibility of cooking, serving, and cleaning up still fell on me and I wanted it this way. I still wanted to preserve my role in life after having lost so much else."

Some research has indicated that couples cope more easily when the woman, rather than the man, is the patient. This is more consistent with conventional roles; the woman can vent her feelings while the man remains strong and stoical (Sales, Schultz, & Biegel, 1992). However, the male partners often have even stronger fears than do their wives. One study of families affected by breast cancer found that the husbands were more fearful of their wives' dying than the wives were and that the husbands manifested a variety of strong reactions including fear, feeling displaced by cancer, denial, and burying themselves in their work (Cullinan, 1992).

The reactions of male partners to cancer has been described as bimodal (Carter & Carter, 1994). Some men withdraw and become distant, uncommunicative, and depressed. These men typically are terrified of abandonment and seem to benefit most from individual counseling. Their partners' withdrawal may be particularly painful for survivors. As one woman wrote, "A real chasm has developed between my husband and me. His disinterest in learning anything about cancer and his insistence that everything was okay struck me as being uncaring and insensitive. I feel I can no longer discuss anything of importance with him."

Although some men distance themselves from the cancer survivor, other men become overprotective and assume responsibility for decisions about the partner's medical treatment. Both patterns seem to reflect prior issues, early loss for the former group and previous patterns of caretaking for the latter group.

Other dimensions of the couple relationship also affect their response to cancer. Couples with matching communication styles (for example, both use denial extensively or both talk very openly) report the least distress related to dealing with illness (McDaniel, Hepworth, & Doherty, 1992). Couples with strong marriages usually handle most stages of cancer better than couples with difficult marriages but may suffer more if the disease becomes terminal. Younger spouses, particularly women, generally have more difficulty dealing with their partner's cancer than do older couples, probably because the disease has struck at an unexpected time and because the woman may fear being left a widow with young children. On the other hand, older partners, particularly those with their own medical concerns as well as those with economic difficulties, are more likely to feel over-whelmed and depressed by the demands placed on them by their partner's illness (Sales, Schultz, & Biegel, 1992).

If cancer and its treatment have caused physical changes or have affected the capacity for intimacy or reproduction, the couple's sexual relationship may be adversely affected. Sexual difficulties usu-ally surface early, generally will be evident within three or four months of cancer treatments (Beckham & Godding, 1990), and may be long-lasting. Burbie and Polinsky (1992) found that 50 per-cent of sexually active women continued to have sexual difficulties eight years after they were treated for breast cancer. Changes in body image may lead to heightened sensitivity, and any sign of rejection may be extremely painful and have serious consequences for the couple relationship. As one woman who had breast cancer said, "When I asked my husband right after the surgery if he wanted to see the scars, he said no, he never wanted to see them. This was devastating to my self-esteem. I had such a feeling of sadness. I knew the marriage was over then."

Helping Couples Cope with Cancer

Psychotherapy for couples dealing with cancer can facilitate adjust-ment and be of long-term benefit to the relationship. Christensen (1983), for example, found that structured couples' counseling fol-lowing the wife's mastectomy, using discussion of the relationship, education, suggestion, role play, behavioral interventions, and attention to self-image, reduced emotional distress and depression and increased sexual satisfaction for both partners. Hopwood and Maguire (1992) concluded that couples who could successfully negotiate role changes, collaborated in decisions regarding treat-ment of cancer, and felt understood were less at risk of developing serious emotional difficulties.

Therapists counseling couples affected by cancer should seek to understand not only the immediate problems of the disease and its treatment but also the previous strengths and weaknesses of the relationship. Previous difficulties may be compounded by cancer and may worsen under pressure, whereas couples with strong relationships may become even stronger in their efforts to fight cancer. One cancer survivor wrote, "My spouse and I were close before; after cancer, we became closer than I would have ever believed."

Promoting communication probably is the first step to helping couples cope with cancer. Even if couples are aware of each other's feelings, pretence awareness is a common response to cancer in which both partners pretend the problems and issues are not there and suppress any negative feelings to avoid upsetting the partner (Cullinan, 1992). Both partners need to talk about the disease and the thoughts and emotions it has brought up for them. While not all thoughts need to be communicated, identification of areas that people do not wish to discuss, as well as the reasons for their decisions, will at least make any withholding less threatening and more acceptable (Rolland, 1994). With open communication, couples can collaborate more easily on making decisions about treatment and family responsibilities. Open communication will also point up any cognitive distortions or misunderstandings that can then be addressed.

Clear communication is also essential to helping couples deal with issues of sexuality. A partner's avoidance of intimacy may reflect a fear of hurting or pressuring the cancer survivor; however, the survivor may interpret this as a rejection or lack of interest. Intimacy should be viewed as involving more than intercourse, and couples can be helped to maintain a sense of closeness even if some sexual activities are not possible. Planning activities that promote sharing and contact but are not too taxing for the survivor, such as a meal at a favorite restaurant, can preserve the closeness of the relationship before cancer and remind couples that cancer need not take over their lives completely. As one man wrote, "We were so caught up in just getting from day to day for so long that we didn't realize the toll it was taking on us and our relationship."

For couples coping with forms of cancer that are disfiguring or that affect the reproductive system or are likely to have an impact on sexuality, Beckham and Godding (1990) recommended preventive interventions as early as possible to reduce or prevent sexual difficulties. Therapists might inquire directly about changes in sexuality as well as about the presence of such symptoms as loss of desire, pain, feeling unattractive, premature menopause, vaginal dryness, or problems with erection even if couples do not present those concerns. Embarrassment and fear of upsetting the partner may prevent people from bring up these difficulties in therapy.

In order to facilitate open communication about these and other difficult areas, therapists probably should have both individual and couples sessions. Areas that are brought up in the individual sessions but not the couples sessions can then be explored and ways to share them with the partner can be developed. Individual meetings also can ensure that different needs and agendas are addressed. Fuller and Swenson (1992), for example, found that for the cancer survivor, affiliation with the spouse had the highest correlation with quality of life whereas coping with problems had the highest correlation with quality of life for the partner.

In addition to improving their communication, most couples will have to establish new patterns of adaptation in order to regain equilibrium. Cognitive and behavioral interventions such as those described in Chapters Five and Six may be useful to family members as well as cancer survivors. Practical help such as time management, decision making, and assertiveness training to enable family members to ask others for assistance can also be very useful. Couples group therapy, with others who are coping with cancer, can be particularly helpful in exposing people to new ways of dealing with problems and new models of family functioning (Knakal, 1988). The group also can provide useful support and information.

Viewing the disease as an outside force having an impact on a relationship can normalize its impact and provide support and a sense of direction and control. While it is important for the couple to work as a team to manage the impact of the disease, their individuality also must be maintained. The partner and if possible the survivor need to have contacts and activities that provide a respite from dealing with cancer and allow them to maintain previous interests as much as possible. One man thought that he should stay with his wife while she slept for thirty six hours following chemotherapy. As a result, he gave up many of his own friends and activities and was becoming resentful. However, discussion made clear that his wife did not need him to be present and in fact felt less guilty herself if her husband took advantage of this time for himself. By having both partners articulate their wants and feelings and by maintaining some separateness, support can be maintained while dependency and enmeshment can be avoided.

The Impact of Cancer in a Family with Children

Cancer can affect children in several ways. Children themselves may be diagnosed with cancer or the children may have a close relative, a parent or sibling, with cancer. This section will look at the impact of cancer on children in the context of their families.

Children with Cancer

Approximately one child in three thousand will be diagnosed with cancer (Macaskill & Monach, 1990). Improvements in medical knowledge have led to dramatic increases in survival rates for children who have had cancer and to an increase in the number of people with a childhood history of cancer. Nevertheless, the death rate from childhood cancer is still about 30 percent (Bertolone & Scott, 1990). Families with children who have cancer may face the following hurdles:

- The diagnosis, the often painful and aggressive treatments, and the immediate threat to the child and the family.
- The fear of recurrence.
- The sometimes permanent changes caused by cancer and its treatment. Some of these, like infertility, amputation of a limb, and impairment of growth and learning, will have a profound impact on the rest of the child's life as well as on the future of the family and may necessitate long-term medical and psychological help.
- The death of the child.

Most children handle cancer treatments better if they have some understanding of what is going on and are less frightened if parents are present (Sitarz, 1990). Consequently, clear communication and cooperation among parents, children, and medical staff can make an important difference in the child's physical and emotional response to cancer and its treatment.

Impact on the Parents

Cancer in a child is an extremely difficult challenge for most families. This diagnosis typically is shocking and unexpected, filling parents with fear, guilt, and helplessness as they watch their child undergo painful and sometimes futile treatments. Parents' initial reaction to the diagnosis of cancer in a child has been described as anticipatory mourning; they may assume the child will die even if the prognosis is encouraging (Macaskill & Monach, 1990).

The process of coping with cancer in a child puts considerable strain on the marital relationship and may lead to marital conflict if parents are not able to share their feelings and work together to navigate this crisis. Although the couple will usually cope with cancer as well or as poorly as they have coped with other stressors they have encountered, even high-functioning families can benefit from some help in dealing with this very difficult crisis. With help, the experience of coping with cancer can strengthen a family. It can draw them closer, lead them to appreciate the family even more, instill pride about the way the family handled the disease, and promote greater responsibility and maturity in the children.

Therapists can help parents of children with cancer in several ways. They need the opportunity to express their feelings, especially their fears. Sometimes husband and wife manage their feelings differently, with the wife typically being more open about her fear and sadness. This difference may lead the couple to devalue and misunderstand each others' feelings, perhaps viewing one style of managing feelings as more appropriate or caring. Therapists can help couples to normalize and address these differences and recognize that even very deep and painful feelings may be expressed in different ways.

The parents usually will need help in managing unrealistic fears and concerns. They may blame themselves for the child's cancer and for minor past transgressions against the person with cancer. They may feel angry and rant against the injustice they have experienced or they may suffer in silence. They may not believe the physician's reassurances, perhaps because of their own self-doubts or a family history of deaths due to cancer. Therapists can help parents to formulate their questions and educate themselves about their child's prognosis and treatment so that they develop realistic expectations about the future. Teaching parents a systematic approach to decision making is another way to help them obtain the information they need and make treatment and other decisions. Cognitive restructuring also may be useful to families who have exaggerated worries.

Parents also need help in becoming a cohesive and effective team. Especially if other children are at home, the couple will have many demands that need attention. They may be making unrealistic demands of themselves as well as of each other. They are likely to need help in organizing their time, in sharing tasks, and in making good use of their support systems. Although the demands of dealing with cancer may seem overwhelming, parents still need to find time to pay attention to their own relationship and to the needs of their other children. Unless that is done, cancer in a child has been found to aggravate existing problems within a marital relationship (Macaskill & Monach, 1990).

Making use of outside supports is an important determinant of parents' adjustment to cancer in a child. Speechley and Noh (1992) found that parents of children with cancer who perceived themselves as having low levels of support were significantly more depressed and anxious and had less marital satisfaction than parents of healthy children; this was not true of parents of children with cancer who believed they did have adequate support. Without adequate support, parents may have difficulty taking care of themselves and setting limits on how much they can do. As a result, they may jeopardize their own health and functioning.

Parents who are employed at the time of the diagnosis may feel torn between their professional demands and those of the family. Focusing total attention on the disease may be counterproductive. Macaskill and Monach (1990) found that parents who continued in their jobs viewed them as a welcome respite from the stress of dealing with cancer. Maintaining other interests and involvements can help parents feel renewed and able to cope with cancer more successfully. Parents without outside commitments might be encouraged to take some time for themselves; people who have no respite from the demands of cancer have been found to have more emotional difficulties. In general, maintaining a normal routine as much as possible is reassuring to all family members.

One concern that most parents have is how much to tell the child with cancer and the other children in the family. Open family communication about the disease, along with mutual support, have been shown to be important factors for positive long-term psychosocial adjustment of children who are cancer survivors (Macaskill & Monach, 1990). Even children as young as three years of age can comprehend the seriousness of their condition and want to talk about it (Sitarz, 1990). Secrecy seems to intensify children's depression and isolation and worsens their fantasies of what is happening to them. Therapists can help parents plan how to tell their children about the disease and decisions that have been made, to encourage their expression of feelings and questions, and to express their own feelings to their children in ways that are reassuring rather than frightening. Also important is giving children a sense of security, support, importance, and belonging, regardless of what stressors are affecting the family.

Overprotection and overindulgence of the cancer survivor is a common issue. Parents may believe they have little time left with the child and so may hover over the child, granting every wish. This may actually be frightening rather than rewarding to the child and certainly can alienate siblings. Especially for adolescents with cancer, parental overprotection may feel suffocating and may lead to conflict. Parents should continue to have reasonable and age-appropriate goals, expectations, and limits for all their children.

Parental attitude can also have an impact on the child's reaction to the cancer treatments. Gorfinkle and Redd (1993) wrote of a feedback loop in which parents who are calm, soothing, and empathic yet distracting while a child is undergoing treatment can help their children manage fears and pain associated with the treatment.

Many hospital and cancer centers have family support groups available. Parents should be encouraged to visit one or more of these groups in an effort to find one that is right for their family and that offers them a place to share and listen and to receive support and information.

The needs of the parents do not end with the end of the treatment. Leventhal-Belfer, Bakker, and Russo (1993) studied parents of childhood cancer survivors an average of eleven years after the diagnosis. Although the group did not have significant psychopathology, most still had pervasive concerns about the health and development of their children and wanted continued support and education. Many of the parents reported it had been very beneficial to share their concerns with their spouse or with friends, but many, particularly the mothers, still wanted contact with other parents who shared their experiences and concerns.

Impact on the Siblings

Siblings too are very much affected by cancer and its treatment. According to McDaniel, Hepworth, and Doherty (1992, p. 222), "Siblings are often the neglected figures in families of chronically ill children." They may fear losing a beloved brother or sister, are scared by the upheaval and upset that has ensued in the family, may worry that they too will develop cancer, may feel jealous or angry at the attention that is being given to the cancer survivor, and may feel guilt about those feelings of jealousy. They may feel pressure to be obedient and responsible and to avoid making demands on the family. Other symptoms often observed in siblings of cancer survivors include irritability and social withdrawal, depression, academic difficulties, regression, enuresis, acting-out behavior, and feelings of loneliness and isolation. Siblings may withdraw from the cancer survivor out of fear of the changes in that person or out of fear of contagion, believing they might contract the disease through contact. The siblings may worry about their own health, may become fearful of physicians, and may even develop somatic symptoms. A common pattern is for the sibling to lose confidence as the sick child gains confidence (Macaskill & Monach, 1990). All of these physical and emotional symptoms are particularly likely to appear if the siblings lack clear information to explain what has happened to the sick child and why the parents' attitudes and behaviors have changed. Without adequate information, siblings tend to feel excluded and rejected, blaming themselves for the changes in the family.

Dealing with problems presented by the siblings of the cancer survivor may be especially difficult for parents; they may feel angry that the siblings do not understand that all the parents' time and attention must be given to the child with cancer. Support systems, especially extended family, may be helpful, giving time and attention to the siblings to compensate for time they have lost with their parents.

Contact between siblings and the cancer survivor should be encouraged. Even if visits or telephone calls are not possible, having the siblings send notes, drawings, or small gifts to the person with cancer can enable them to feel involved and helpful.

Expressive therapy, using drawing, music, or puppets, can be very helpful to siblings. They may be reluctant to verbalize their feelings and reactions directly but may be more open when indirect and creative forms of self-expression are used.

Group counseling can be useful to siblings of children with cancer. This may take the form of support groups at school, groups offered through a cancer treatment facility or a mental health center, or family camps for children with cancer and their siblings. One effective model is a hospital-based peer support and therapy group for children with cancer and their siblings (Jensen, 1990). Children between the ages of eight and eighteen were divided into groups of fifteen to twenty members in which half had been diagnosed with cancer and half were their siblings. Drawing in response to suggested topics and storytelling helped the children express and work through their feelings. In addition, visualization and relaxation skills were taught to help the children with cancer manage their treatments as well as to help their siblings understand and feel a part of the process.

Parents Who Have Cancer: Impact on Children and Adolescents

Perhaps even more frightening to a child than a sibling with cancer is a parent with cancer. Especially for young children who may view their parents as all-powerful and invulnerable, the threat of losing a parent, as well as the physical changes caused by cancer and its treatment, may be terrifying to the child.

Children's reactions to cancer in a parent may be affected by many factors that should be explored. If the relationship has been a conflicted one, children may feel guilty and may distance themselves from their parents. Sadness may be particularly acute in close relationships, and even these children may withdraw because seeing the parent is so painful. If the child is already troubled or in a difficult or transitional stage such as adolescence, dealing with cancer may compound those difficulties and lead to considerable emotional turmoil. The type of cancer seems to affect the children's responses. Sales, Schultz, and Biegel (1992) reported that daughters were especially supportive of their mothers with breast cancer while sons had more difficulty dealing with their mothers' breast cancer, perhaps because of its sexual and personal associations.

Greening (1992) identified five needs of young children with a parent who has cancer: (1) clear information, (2) feeling involved and important, (3) reassurance, (4) opportunity to express their thoughts and feelings, and (5) maintenance of their usual interests and activities. Open, clear communication, affording children the opportunity to ask questions and express their feelings about their parents' illness, seems most important to their adjustment. However, children are often reluctant to burden their parents with their fears because they do not want to upset them; thus, they may withhold their reactions to their parents' illness and act as if they are coping well. In reality, they are likely to be struggling with anxiety and depression and may not be functioning well at school or with friends.

Peer support groups that afford children the opportunity to share their experiences with others who understand can be very helpful. In that context, most children seem able to express honestly the fears and emotions they may be unwilling to share with the parents. Groups are also useful in normalizing feelings, reducing stigma, and preserving age-appropriate ties and interests. If such a group cannot be found, individual or family sessions with a psychotherapist are a good alternative, providing children a setting in which it is safe for them to express their worst fears.

A model for a group intervention for children whose parents have cancer was developed by Taylor-Brown, Acheson, and Farber (1993). Their program, Kids Can Cope, was designed for children between the ages of five and eighteen. Goals included providing information on cancer and its treatment, an opportunity to share feelings in a safe environment, improvement in the children's repertoire of effective coping skills, support, and development of a positive perception of the medical staff. Six sessions were held, with four to eight members of similar ages in each group. Session 1 focused on building trust and cohesion and assessing the children's needs. Session 2 provided education on cancer and on people's emotional reactions to the disease. Sessions 3 and 4 provided the children an opportunity to express and explore their feelings while sessions 5 and 6 focused on developing their coping skills. Therapists sought to normalize feelings, to clarify misconceptions about the disease, and to encourage the children to communicate openly with their parents. The youngest children were most concerned about the impact of the disease on the parent with cancer and on their family. The children in early adolescence focused more on how cancer affected them personally and on issues of responsibility and independence.

A similar group experience, the Bear Essentials program, was developed for younger children, ages four to eight, and their parents (Greening, 1992). That program made greater use of hands-on activities, music, puppets, crafts such as making masks to show feelings, and cards and gifts for the parents. The group meetings seemed to reduce confusion and isolation and helped to empower and strengthen the families.

Reading about cancer and its impact on families can also help children understand what is happening and can normalize their reactions. Bernstein and Rudman (1989) developed a useful annotated bibliography of books that can help children deal with illness, separation, and loss.

Parents Who Have Cancer: Their Own Struggle

Parents facing the possible loss of their families, as well as their lives, of course, are also prone to have difficulty in their family relationships. Parents may pressure or spoil their children, fearing that they have little time left with them and wanting to do all they can to ensure their children's future success. Single parents are particularly prone to this pattern (Rolland, 1994). This may lead the children to withdraw or become angry at the parent at a time when the parent is emotionally and physically vulnerable and may be confused and hurt by the child's reaction. Parents may need help in understanding the impact of cancer on their children and in realizing that reactions in their children such as anger, embarrassment, and denial are common and normal.

Parents often need help in planning how to talk with their children about cancer. Parents should avoid giving children false reassurance but also should be gentle and encouraging. In response to the question of whether a parent is going to die, the parent might respond, "I'm doing very well. I'm getting good treatment and the doctors are doing everything possible to help me have a very long life." Parents also can help by anticipating children's emotional reactions, encouraging them to continue their usual activities, giving them a helpful role to play in dealing with cancer, providing information and support, adding a new focus to the child's life, and maintaining a regular routine and a predictable schedule as much as possible.

Parents may feel shocked by some of their own reactions. A woman with breast cancer, for example, may feel envious of her adolescent daughter's health and attractiveness. These feelings too can be normalized as therapists let cancer survivors know that all feelings can be expressed during psychotherapy. Parents can be helped to acknowledge their own concerns and feelings without overwhelming or burdening their children with frightening images and ideas.

Parents Who Have Cancer: Impact on Adult Children

Adult children too may have difficulty dealing with cancer in a parent. In addition to the issue of loss of a loved one, several other issues often arise. Particularly if the parent-child bond has been a close one and the adult child is the same gender and much like the parent in appearance and behavior, the adult child may worry about genetic transmission of the disease and may fear that he or she will develop cancer in the future. Adult children of cancer survivors may view a parent's illness as a preview of what they expect to happen to them and that may make dealing with the disease particularly painful.

The diagnosis of cancer may necessitate a role reversal, in which the adult child assumes care of the parent. For most adult children who have their own family and career responsibilities, this can feel burdensome and difficult. This is especially true of adult children who have felt estranged or in conflict with their parents and for adult children who may be pressured into the caretaking role because of gender or other family expectations (the oldest child or the wife of the closest son). Dealing with cancer can be very difficult and upsetting whenever it threatens the parent-child bond. Therapists should keep this in mind when counseling families affected by cancer.

The Impact of Cancer on Friendships

Cancer affects all relationships: those with friends and colleagues as well as those with family members. The importance of support systems has been discussed elsewhere in this book. Many cancer survivors look beyond their families and seek support as well as practical help from friends and associates.

Unfortunately, responses to cancer survivors vary. Some friends reach out to the survivor and the process of seeing a friend through cancer and its treatment can lead to a deepening of the relationship. On the other hand, many people avoid the cancer survivor and what little contact is made is uncomfortable and even hurtful. In the words of cancer survivors, "I'm bald, nauseous, scarred, and weak. My very presence makes others uncomfortable. . . . Suddenly people I'd known all my life felt awkward in communicating with me. . . . I lost one friend because he couldn't cope with the fact that I had cancer. He kept saying, 'I'm sure you'll be just fine.'"

Although of course cancer survivors should not be held responsible for their friends' discomfort with their disease, certain behaviors on the part of cancer survivors may increase the discomfort experienced by their friends and associates. Some survivors overwhelm others with their need to express their feelings: "I told just about everyone all the details of my cancer and its treatment. I believe I was in shock and kept needing to say I had cancer in order to believe it myself." Other cancer survivors avoid people or give the message that they do not need any help because of their own self-consciousness about their disease. As one cancer survivor said, "How do you gracefully tell someone that you've had cancer and that even hugs hurt? It was easier for me to just stay home with my husband and avoid other people." This reaction is understandable, but it puts a great deal of pressure on immediate family members who may become the cancer survivor's only source of support. It may also deny friends the opportunity for the involvement they would like to have with the survivor.

Psychotherapists can help cancer survivors to look at their feelings about telling others that they have cancer. They may fear that others will think they are contagious, will pity or blame them, will be revolted by them, will believe their death is inevitable, or will view them as complaining or self-indulgent. Cognitive-behavioral approaches can help people assess the reality of these concerns and plan ways to tell people about the disease that minimize the likelihood of a negative reaction.

Most people who do shy away from cancer survivors seem to do so out of discomfort and lack of information on how to help. Some of those negative reactions can be offset if cancer survivors give people clear information on what they need, whether it is just visiting and talking or practical help such as transportation, child care, meal preparation, or companionship during a treatment procedure. Cancer survivors should also be encouraged to ask about reactions and feelings of their friends and associates; giving them an opportunity to talk about their own feelings may reduce their fears and embarrassment. If friends manifest behaviors that are not helpful, such as telling stories about people who have died of cancer, the survivors should be encouraged to verbalize their discomfort and indicate what would be more helpful to them. Role playing or rehearsal in a therapy session, as well as attention to communication and assertiveness skills, can help people express themselves more directly to others.

Cancer survivors also benefit from help in returning to work or encountering friends and neighbors. They may not know who is aware that they had cancer, may fear discrimination and stigmatization in the workplace, and may worry that people will treat them differently. These fears are sometimes realistic. Although therapists cannot prevent these negative responses, they can help cancer survivors to anticipate them and plan ways to deal with them so they will not feel confused or caught off guard.

One man, a teacher, learned that rumors had circulated among other teachers and students that he was dying. In reality, he had an excellent prognosis. Rather than wondering what people were thinking, he decided to take control of the situation when he returned to work and announced in his classes as well as at a faculty meeting that he had been treated for cancer, had an excellent prognosis, and expected to live a long life. This ended most of the gossiping and enabled him to resume his work with fewer worries.

Children with cancer who are returning to school may have considerable difficulty both with their classmates' reactions and their own feelings of shame and concern about changes in their appearance. Friends may withdraw from or tease cancer survivors as well as their siblings. Parents should inform teachers and school counselors of their child's situation and enlist their help in facilitating the child's return to the classroom. In addition, children may be helped by anticipating both positive and negative reactions they may receive and developing responses or coping mechanisms, including seeking help from adults.

The Impact of Cancer on Special Populations

Although cancer inevitably has an impact on relationships and support systems, that impact may be particularly difficult for people in certain gender or psychosocial groups, including the following (Haber, 1993):

Men typically have more difficulty than women in seeking support and in telling others about their disease.

People from low socioeconomic groups or ethnic minorities have lower survival rates for some types of cancer. This may be due to many factors including their difficulty in negotiating the bureaucracy of medical treatment and insurance, their limited access to support systems, their heightened family and financial responsibilities, and their own misinformation about cancer.

Gay men and lesbians may face discrimination from the health care system as well as limitations on hospital visits from people to whom they are not related. They may experience discomfort about informing others of their sexual orientation and so may not give physicians accurate information about the important role their partners play in their lives.

Older people may have limited social and financial resources and may not be familiar with the availability and importance of support groups. They may have grown up at a time when cancer generally was not discussed and when the prognosis was far worse than it is now. Those attitudes may prevent them from telling others of their disease and from having an accurate understanding of their prognosis.

Therapists should be sure to view their clients who are cancer survivors in context, considering their available support systems, their history of using support systems, and their own attitudes that may interfere with their receiving the support they need. Enabling people to overcome barriers to support and assistance, while respecting their styles and preferences, can help even isolated clients find appropriate support systems.

Overview of Chapter

Most families have the resources they need to cope with cancer and do not need extensive or intensive psychotherapy. At the same time, most families seem to benefit from some short-term, supportive counseling that helps them to understand and manage the impact cancer is having on their family, to share their feelings and listen to each other in a safe place, to maintain their usual routine as much as possible, to communicate with and make good use of their support systems, and to deal with cancer in a way that is likely to be beneficial to the cancer survivor as well as to the family. This chapter has provided information to help therapists work more effectively with the friends and family of cancer survivors and to help survivors obtain the help they need from their families and friends.

10

· ·

Relationships with Treatment Providers

The relationship between cancer survivors and the professionals who seek to help them is an important ingredient not only of cancer survivors' attitude toward and adjustment to cancer but also of their prognosis. Obtaining clear and accurate information on their condition, making sound treatment decisions, and having the motivation to comply with difficult treatments can make an important difference in the health of cancer survivors. This chapter looks at the interactions between cancer survivors and their health care providers and what survivors as well as therapists can do to facilitate that interaction. This chapter also explores the role of psychotherapists who work with cancer survivors and issues that may arise in that relationship. Because research on these topics is very limited, I will draw more heavily than in the other chapters on my own experiences in working with cancer survivors.

The Importance of Medical Information

The diagnosis of cancer is a shocking blow to most people. Before they have much time to recover from that shock, they must make decisions that will have a profound impact on their lives and those of people close to them. Some cancer survivors become immobilized by this experience and turn these decisions over to a physician or loved one. Other cancer survivors assume as much control as they can of the situation; they research their disease, obtain multiple medical opinions, and talk to other cancer survivors so that they know their options and can make an informed decision. Although not all people have the knowledge or interest in such assertive information gathering, having adequate information and clearly formulated questions can take some of the fear out of cancer and its treatment and can lead to better decisions. Studies have also shown that giving people full information about their medical condition results in much less depression and need for psychotropic medications than giving little or no information (Breitbart, 1990). This is consistent with the findings discussed in Chapter One of this book that showed a connection between assertiveness, expressiveness, and involvement on the one hand and a positive prognosis for cancer on the other.

Cancer Survivors and Health Care Providers

People with cancer are usually treated by a group of medical personnel. Initially, a physician who might specialize in gynecology, urology, or general medicine suspects the presence of cancer. That person makes a referral to an oncologist and/or surgeon to confirm the diagnosis. A specialist in reconstructive surgery may join the team, along with a specialist in radiotherapy. Each of these five physicians will have assistants. Oncologists usually are the key people in the medical team; however, their availability may be limited by their busy schedules, emergencies, and their own reluctance to develop close ties to people who are dealing with life-threatening illnesses. The oncologist will have nurses who usually play a primary role in the administration of chemotherapy. Medical technicians will be involved in drawing blood, taking X rays, and providing other tests and scans. Technicians also play an active role in daily radiotherapy treatments. Not surprisingly, many cancer survivors have difficulty figuring out what questions should be directed to each person.

Reactions to Health Care Providers

Cancer survivors inevitably have strong reactions to their health care team as can be seen from the following statements of cancer survivors. Some are positive: "My doctor explained it all and answered questions. When he said attitude played a big role in the success of the treatments, I knew I had a very good chance." However, many are negative:

"Doctors were cold and indifferent. They didn't even introduce themselves."

"My questions to my doctors go unanswered because I'm told I might misinterpret the facts. In reality, knowledge can add to my strength."

"When I react with despair and tears, I'm sedated, threatened with hospitalization, or ignored."

"My internist of seventeen years calmly shook my hand and told me to find a different doctor. It was as if I had become a hideous disease instead of a person."

"Doctors can be very hurtful when they don't want to answer your questions, when they are impatient, when they don't listen, when money seems more important than your life, when they don't believe in you, and when they don't give you their best shot."

Although some of these people may have misunderstood their physicians' motives, what comes across to many cancer survivors is a callous disinterest on the part of their physicians. Physicians may have little or no training in helping people deal with the emotional impact of cancer and may not view that as an appropriate part of their role. As one oncologist told me, "If I got involved with all my patients' personal problems, I couldn't get my job done." The burden then is on cancer survivors to find ways to communicate effectively with their health care providers and obtain the information and support they need.

A positive relationship with medical staff can affect prognosis as well as emotional adjustment. Levy et al. (1990) found that natural killer cell activity was positively associated with a perception of high-quality emotional support from one's physician (as well as from one's partner) in women with early-stage breast cancer. According to one person with cancer, "The people who are survivors don't just accept but ask for information and turn the process around to participate in their own health care."

Improving Patient-Physician Communication

A series of steps can improve patient-physician communication, the trust cancer survivors have in their medical care, and even the quality of that care:

1. *Select physicians carefully.* This is critical to developing good communication with the health care team. Cancer survivors should be encouraged to seek information on the credentials, experience, and specializations of their physicians and to use that information as well as recommendations from other physicians and cancer survivors in making their choices. Cancer survivors should also trust their own reactions to a physician. Particularly when it comes to selecting an oncologist, survivors should be sure they are comfortable with the person's communication style. The oncologist will oversee the treatment process and will be an important figure in the life of the cancer survivor for many years.

Convenience and ambience of the medical setting are other important factors, particularly for people receiving daily radiotherapy treatments or frequent chemotherapy that may cause nausea and discomfort. Most large cities have cancer treatment centers that house all members of an oncology team in the same facility. However, such facilities sometimes seem overwhelming, impersonal, and frightening. Some people may prefer the efficient and impersonal quality of such a center while others may find the office of a private oncologist to be more comfortable.

2. *Gather adequate information.* Some cancer survivors put great time and effort into this process: "I researched my cancer and kept a journal of questions and observations to discuss at doctor's visits.

It worked very well." Therapists can help survivors to become well informed by exploring with them what they already know about their disease and what gaps there are in their information. These gaps can then be formulated into questions, written down, and plans made for when and how to obtain the information. However, the information-gathering process should be tailored to the individual and should consider how much information a person is comfortable receiving and how that person prefers to obtain information.

Information is available from many sources. The American Cancer Society as well as other organizations can be contacted for information on cancer and its treatments (see Resources section at the back of this book). Medical, university, and general libraries are excellent sources of information for people who are comfortable using those resources. People may request copies of their laboratory reports, may ask that specific tests be done on tissue from their tumors, and may request that their slides be sent to a nationally known cancer center for a second opinion. Many first-person accounts written by people who are cancer survivors are available in bookstores, and other cancer survivors are an excellent source of information, particularly on coping with cancer treatments and their side effects. Of course, oncologists and other members of the medical team will probably be the primary source of information.

Some cancer survivors are reluctant to ask their physicians many questions. The survivors may not want to "waste the time of the busy physicians," they may believe their concerns are unimportant or unrealistic, or they may fear that the medical staff will dislike them or view them as complaining or difficult. Therapists should explore internal as well as external barriers to communication with medical staff and should help cancer survivors develop the skills and confidence they need to ask their questions. Role playing as well as writing scripts can help people formulate questions in clear, direct ways that minimize their use of physicians' time.

3. *Process information effectively.* Cancer survivors typically receive a great deal of information from a variety of sources. Some

of this information may be transmitted under stressful conditions, such as immediately after the diagnosis has been confirmed. Retaining and understanding this information may be a challenge for the cancer survivor. This process can be facilitated if survivors bring a companion to important medical appointments to help them ask necessary questions and recall the information. Physicians generally recommend that patients bring another person with them to the consultation and approximately three-fourths of cancer survivors do so (Beisecker & Moore, 1994). Physicians have been found to give more time and information to cancer patients when they are accompanied by a family member, although the physician may actually be less supportive, probably because the person already has a support system present (Labrecque, Blanchard, Ruckdeschel, & Blanchard, 1991). In addition, bringing a companion to medical consultations raises the possibility of two-against-one coalitions, conflicting agendas between the cancer survivor and the companion, and the companion's taking too much control of the meeting. Therapists should keep these dynamics in mind when discussing with a cancer survivor whether to bring a companion to medical consultations and who that companion should be.

Some people bring a tape recorder to their medical appointments as another way to ensure that they hear information accurately. Many cancer survivors benefit from keeping a notebook in which they list medical appointments and sources of help and information, record their questions before each medical consultation, and then write down the answers as well as other important information. Reviewing this information later in a relaxed context can help them absorb what has been said and make good use of the information.

Physicians are not always pleased with the time-consuming questions and participation in decision making evidenced by some cancer survivors. Temoshok and Dreher (1992) described some cancer survivors with a fighting spirit as "too mean to die" (p. 130). Therapists can help their clients present questions and requests in assertive rather than aggressive ways. At the same time, cancer survivors and therapists should be prepared for some physicians to react negatively to healthy and self-empowering behaviors on the part of cancer survivors.

4. *Making sound decisions.* What is the stage of my cancer and how was that determined? What are my treatment options? How will each treatment affect my prognosis? What are the likely benefits and problems associated with each treatment option? What would you recommend and why? These and other key questions can help cancer survivors make necessary decisions about the treatment of their disease as well as about other areas of their lives.

Common decisions focus on what medical tests to use to clarify the nature of the disease, whether to participate in clinical trials of treatments that are promising but not yet standard procedure, whether to have surgery, whether and what types of reconstructive surgery to select, whether to have chemotherapy and if so what type of chemotherapy, whether to have radiotherapy, whether to have hormone treatments, and in what order treatments should be provided. Different opinions and uncertainty are common in cancer treatment, and percentages may be the most definitive information that can be provided. One cancer survivor, for example, was told that her prognosis was 20 percent with surgery alone, 40 percent with the addition of relatively mild chemotherapy, 60 percent with the addition of intensive chemotherapy and radiotherapy, and even higher with a bone marrow transplant, which posed a 10 percent risk of fatality. Based on tentative and complex information, a decision had to be made that seemed right for the woman and her family. Clearly, decisions about cancer treatments often involve considerable ambiguity and stress.

Cancer survivors also need to make decisions about other areas of their lives. They need to know how much help they will need with child care and household responsibilities, if and when they can expect to return to work, what impairment in functioning they are likely to experience, and what their treatments are likely to cost. For some people, cancer is a catalyst that prompts them to make living and traditional wills and to plan for their deaths, even if their prognosis is positive. An attitude of "hope for the best but prepare for the worst" seems both realistic and reassuring to cancer survivors and can help them move forward with difficult plans and decisions.

Decision making has been discussed in Chapter Five of this book. Using a structured, organized approach to decision making in which the options and their pros and cons are explored and weighed can help people to feel a sense of control over the process of dealing with cancer and can result in sound decisions that people will be motivated to implement.

The Psychotherapist as Liaison with the Health Care Team

Therapists can facilitate patient-physician communication by establishing contact with the physicians. McDaniel, Hepworth, and Doherty (1992) suggested inviting a physician to a joint therapy session with the client. Although few physicians' schedules may accommodate such meetings, other possible ways to meet include the therapist accompanying the client to a medical consultation or, as I have experienced, a physician meeting with a support group that included many of his patients as well as their therapist.

Of course, psychotherapists should only establish contact with physicians with the cancer survivor's approval and written permission for therapist and physician to exchange information. In cases where I have communicated directly with physicians, it has always resulted in the physicians treating the clients with more compassion and sensitivity, answering their questions more fully, improving the patient-physician rapport, and giving cancer survivors a greater sense of empowerment. Psychotherapist-physician communication can also give the encouraging message that cancer survivors, their family, the health care providers, and the psychotherapist all are part of a team that is doing its best to restore the patients' health. However, issues of confidentiality, territoriality, and busy schedules should be handled carefully so that they do not prevent establishment of a collaboration between medical and psychosocial treatment providers.

Poor communication between physicians and patients sometimes stems from misunderstanding of each others' motives and reactions. For example, an oncologist viewed one of my clients as emotionally unstable and provided her as little information as possible to avoid upsetting her. The woman interpreted this as reluctance to give her bad news and became increasingly fearful that her physician was concealing information from her, which caused her to cry during many of her oncology appointments. Her tearfulness was viewed by the oncologist as an indication that he was correct in withholding information. In reality, this was a strong and resourceful woman who craved information. When I explained this to the physician and reassured him that the woman was not at risk of becoming suicidal or psychotic, he gradually became more direct with the woman, and her distress in turn lessened.

Another woman was unable to accurately comprehend information given her by her oncologist because of her high anxiety; that problem was addressed by the therapist becoming a channel of communication. All three agreed that information would not be given directly to the patient but would be transmitted in writing or by telephone to the therapist, who would then provide the information to the cancer survivor. In this way, the therapist could ensure that the woman was correctly understanding the information and had the opportunity to express her feelings in a safe and accepting context. Of course, the therapist could not answer the woman's medical questions, but together they would formulate questions that would then be transmitted to the physician who would provide the answers to the therapist. After a brief period of this approach to communication, the woman became impatient with the process and marshaled the self-confidence to initiate direct contact with the oncologist.

Rights of Cancer Survivors

Another way for therapists to help cancer survivors interact positively with their health care providers is by familiarizing the survivors with their rights and helping them to safeguard those rights. Knowing that they have rights can be comforting and empowering to cancer survivors.

Temoshok and Dreher (1992), Winograd (1992), and others have written about the rights of cancer survivors. The following are important rights:

- The right to have hope

- The right to complete and accurate information

- The right to make their own decisions

- The right to express their emotions and needs and be heard

- The right to respect, privacy, and dignity

- The right to any treatments, medical or psychosocial, that are likely to improve or maintain their health and reduce discomfort

- The right to use psychotherapeutic services as an adjunct to their medical treatments to help them better handle the impact of cancer and its treatment

- The right to maintain closeness with family and friends and to involve them in their decisions and treatments as much as possible

- The right to make the most of each day, to seek and experience joy in their lives for as long as they can

- The right to support and help from professionals, family, and friends

Psychotherapists' Use of Medical Information

Because psychotherapists will be receiving a great deal of medical information from physicians and cancer survivors, they should acquire some knowledge of the medical aspects of cancer and its treatment. According to Haber (1993, p. 10), "Familiarity with medical issues makes it easier for the psychologist to dispel fears, anxieties, and myths and to stay focused on the individual's psychological reaction without becoming distracted or overwhelmed by the medical component." Therapists should be familiar with the major types of cancer, the process of staging cancer and the meaning of the stages, and the nature and side effects of common treatments for cancer. Through their work with cancer survivors, most therapists will become familiar with oncologists, surgeons, and others who provide medical treatment to cancer survivors. This information can enable therapists to provide their clients with some information on cancer and its treatment, to help their clients ask the questions and get the information they need, and to suggest sources of information and medical treatment.

However, possession of medical information on cancer and its treatment also poses several risks. Therapists must be very careful not to take on the role of the physician and of course should not make any medical recommendations to their clients. Therapists may say something like, "Common concerns of people I have counseled who have gone through radiotherapy include . . . " or "For most people, hair loss from chemotherapy happens in the following way . . ." but they should emphasize that each person reacts differently to treatment and the best source of information is the physician.

Sometimes cancer survivors will give the therapist medical information that sounds questionable or unethical. For example, one woman who had a mastectomy following a diagnosis of breast cancer reported that her physician had not removed lymph nodes from surrounding tissue to determine whether the cancer had spread beyond the breast. This violated standard operating procedure but may have been due to some special circumstance unknown to the therapist. Here too therapists must be cautious and must not venture outside of their areas of expertise. On the other hand, to ignore this potential omission would seem hurtful to the client. Again, assuming a tentative stance, therapists might say, "From what I have learned, lymph nodes usually are tested when a mastectomy is performed. Perhaps you would want to ask the physician why that procedure was not done and what information she has on whether your cancer has metastasized?"

A similar situation often arises when addressing the side effects of chemotherapy. Physicians sometimes minimize the potential impact of chemotherapy, perhaps not wanting to frighten someone undergoing treatment. However, this may lead people to worry that a side effect is actually a sign that the cancer has spread. Again, the therapist can provide some information and encourage a medical consultation: "I know your physician didn't tell you that some memory loss and difficulty concentrating may be side effects of chemotherapy, but I have had other people undergoing chemotherapy report those reactions. It may well not mean that the cancer has metastasized to your brain as you believe. I would strongly encourage you to contact your oncologist as soon as possible to discuss these symptoms."

Therapists may also be tempted to provide medical advice when a client makes apparently unsound medical decisions. For example, one cancer survivor intended to miss a week of radiotherapy appointments because they conflicted with a business trip that was important to him. Even in what may seem to be self-destructive decisions like this one, therapists need to allow people to make their own decisions and to respect their autonomy and self-determination. However, therapists might encourage people to try healthier choices for a limited time and then reevaluate their decisions and certainly can explore fully with their clients the consequences of their choices and possible alternatives. In the above situation, arrangements were made for the man to receive his treatments at a hospital in the city he was visiting so that he could take his trip and maintain his treatment schedule.

Although all decisions are the client's, therapists can promote compliance with medical treatment by emphasizing that psychotherapy is an adjunct, not an alternative, to conventional medical treatment; by encouraging people to become involved and active in gathering information and making thoughtful decisions; and by using interventions that help cancer survivors cope effectively with the emotional and physical consequences of their disease and its treatment.

Psychotherapists Working with Cancer Survivors

Whether therapists specialize in counseling cancer survivors or have a general practice, people with cancer as well as people whose family members have cancer inevitably will appear on their caseload. Over 10 percent of all women will be diagnosed with breast cancer in their lifetime and that represents only one of more than 100 types of cancer. One out of four people in the United States and three out of four families will be confronted with cancer in their lifetimes (Schag, Heinrich, & Ganz, 1983).

The field of psychooncology, studying and treating the affective, cognitive, and behavioral difficulties of people with cancer and their families, is a growing specialty and increasing numbers of hospitals and cancer treatment centers include a mental health professional on the staff. Although the basic skills of the psychotherapist are essential to working effectively with cancer survivors as they are with all people, certain skills and areas of knowledge that have been discussed elsewhere in this book are particularly appropriate for use with cancer survivors. In addition, there are special benefits and challenges that come from working with people affected by cancer.

Role of the Therapist

People who have been diagnosed with cancer are going through a life-threatening and urgent situation. For most, this experience will be a crisis in their lives, requiring a great expenditure of their energy and resources. Therapists working with cancer survivors also need to mobilize their energy and resources. Norman and Brandeis (1992) described the interaction of therapist and cancer survivor as an arm-in-arm approach. The importance of establishing a collaborative, trusting relationship based on caring, authenticity, and a mutual goal of coping effectively with cancer cannot be underemphasized. According to Kash and Breitbart (1993, p. 244), "Psychotherapy with cancer patients demands a far more active stance and use of the self than is true of traditional psychotherapy, making the need for self-awareness more important." Flexibility is also important in effective therapy with cancer survivors. Appointment times may need to be changed with little notice due to the cancer survivor's physical condition and treatment requirement; home or hospital visits may be indicated; and collaboration with physicians, hospital social workers, support group leaders, and hospice staff may be part of the therapist's role.

Clients will need rapid and effective assistance in coping with the shock of the diagnosis, making medical and personal decisions, and dealing with the rigors of their treatments. Although of course some attention needs to be paid to gathering background information and viewing the person and the disease in context, the primary focus of treatment will be on the present crisis.

Assuming an active, flexible, and relatively directive stance is needed in order to quickly build adequate rapport and trust and mobilize the coping skills of cancer survivors. In my first session with a cancer survivor, I provide an overview of my approach to therapy, describing some of the cognitive, behavioral, and other techniques that have proven to be effective with cancer survivors and the potential benefits that these tools can bring. I also reassure people that although my focus will be on thoughts and behaviors, expressing and dealing with emotions is also essential to coping with cancer and therapy will allow opportunity for that as well. Finally, I tell my clients that at the end of each session we will agree on one or more tasks for them to do between sessions; this seems to accelerate the therapeutic process and facilitates application of the interventions to the actual process of dealing with cancer and its treatments. Although I respect my clients' defenses, I raise other possibilities if I believe they are acting in self-destructive ways and I will suggest another point of view or behavior and encourage them to discuss alternatives. "What if" can be a useful question to broaden a person's perspective while still supporting optimism: for example, "I hope your treatment will be effective, but what if the cancer continues to spread?"

I try to provide my clients a great deal of support and empathy as they go through their treatments. I will call or give them the option of telephoning me at critical moments such as immediately before and after surgery or their first chemotherapy treatment. Cancer survivors seem to appreciate this; it gives them the message that I am part of the team, along with their physicians, family, and friends, to help them fight cancer. As one client wrote, "It is helpful that on the morning after your surgery, the phone rings and it is your therapist calling to see how you are, to wish you well, and to share your happiness that the strategies we developed together really worked!" Some clinicians have suggested meditating with clients as another way of both teaching people a useful tool and joining with them in a powerful way (Chandler, Holden, & Kolander, 1992). One program, providing hospital-based therapy, arranged to have a counselor present when women who had mastectomies first saw the scar from their surgery (Watson, Denton, Baum, & Greer, 1988). Therapists may also choose to visit their clients in the hospital or to join families at funerals or memorial services. Whatever methods are used, a supportive, active, and interactive approach seems best for promoting an effective and collaborative relationship with cancer survivors.

Language is important in the therapist–cancer survivor relationship. People sometimes use discouraging and misleading language to refer to cancer. For example, cancer may be described as a terminal illness or cancer survivors may be asked shortly after treatment if they are cured. Therapists should carefully monitor their choice of words so that they communicate a realistic optimism. I speak of cancer survivors rather than people with cancer or victims of cancer, and once people begin their treatments and no longer have active signs of the disease, I deliberately use the past tense and talk about when they had cancer or when the disease was diagnosed. Questions should be carefully phrased so that they do not imply survivors are responsible for their disease. Strategies should be presented as ways to cope with cancer, rather than to cure. Realistic hope should be encouraged without providing false reassurance.

Doka (1993) provided a list of criteria for the sensitive caregiver who is working with people with life-threatening illnesses. These offer a useful picture of the multifaceted role of therapists who counsel cancer survivors. According to Doka, such a caregiver needs to be sensitive to the following:

- The whole person

- The person's various roles

- Cultural differences

- Diverse age groups and populations

- The nature and dynamics of families

- The importance of open, mutual communication

- Promoting the independence of the person

- The importance of establishing and moving toward goals

- Problems of pain and discomfort

- The therapist's own role, feelings, wants, and needs

Challenges and Rewards

Counseling cancer survivors can be extremely rewarding. In a relatively brief period of time, therapists can see people who came into therapy feeling depressed, terrified, and overwhelmed become people who are successfully managing a very difficult situation, who have developed a fighting spirit, and who have grown in self-esteem, self-efficacy, and optimism. Family members too usually respond well to treatment. As few as one or two sessions that afford family members and cancer survivors the opportunity to share their feelings, to provide each other support and understanding, and to improve their communication can make a great difference in family members' own adjustment and coping as well as the help they can provide to the survivor.

On the other hand, psychotherapy with cancer survivors can be difficult and emotionally draining. Dealing with issues of death and disability may raise therapists' own feelings of vulnerability and inadequacy (Kash & Breitbart, 1993). Therapists may overemphasize their own importance, believing they are the only ones who really understand the cancer survivor, or they may underemphasize their role, feeling like an outsider who has little to contribute compared to the physicians. Therapists may feel an anxiety-provoking sense of urgency to mobilize people's resources rapidly and may experience a strong wish to save the person from cancer. Their own fears of cancer may be increased along with an exacerbation of feelings of stress.

Therapists working with cancer survivors may experience such negative feelings as a loss of enthusiasm for their work, a sense of discouragement, feelings of depression and burnout, cynicism, tension, irritability, and detachment or overinvolvement in their work. They may have difficulty billing people who are dying and may feel they should not set limits on the frequency and length of sessions they have with seriously ill clients and their families. Colleagues as well as family and friends of therapists working with cancer survivors may avoid discussing their work with them, may view what they do as depressing and unrewarding, may resent the energy they put into their work, or may idealize them in an unrealistic way.

Therapists share with their clients their fears of recurrence and, for some clients, deterioration and death. Therapists too will need to tolerate uncertainty and loss and deal with their own anxieties about cancer, disfigurement, and death. Therapists will grieve with their clients and their family members and will experience their own sense of loss when people with whom they have built a bond do not survive the disease. The recurrences and deaths of children and of clients who resemble the therapist in terms of age, gender, and other variables are likely to be particularly difficult as are losses that are reminiscent of those therapists have experienced in their own lives. Therapists may find themselves becoming tearful or even crying with their clients. As long as the therapist maintains control of the session and keeps the focus on the client, such strong feelings can communicate a great depth of empathy and caring and need not be suppressed.

McEvoy (1990) delineated five stages of grief typically experienced by caregivers who are working with people who are dying. These may be useful for therapists to keep in mind. These stages include the following:

1. Intellectualization (knowledge of the situation, anxiety, withdrawal)
2. Heightened emotions (fear, guilt, confrontation of possibility of own death)
3. Depression (pain, mourning, and grief)
4. Emotional arrival (moderation of feelings, acceptance, realization that one can grieve and then recover)
5. Deep compassion (increase in self-awareness and self-realization, respect and appreciation for the self and the dying person)

Therapists need to establish a fine balance in which they communicate caring and empathy for their clients yet separate themselves from their work enough so they are not impaired or devastated by the loss of some of their clients. They need to engage in life-affirming activities, take care of their own physical and emotional needs, use approaches to stress management and relaxation, and set realistic goals for themselves. They need to be aware of their own responses to potential or actual losses and be able to explore and express their own wants and feelings. Kash and Breitbart (1993) emphasized the importance of therapists who work with cancer survivors maintaining their hardiness, an orientation to life that includes control, commitment, and challenge. Having some balance in their work, seeing clients who are not struggling with cancer as well as those who are, can also help.

In addition, receiving supervision, continuing their own therapy, or participating in peer support groups can be helpful to therapists working with cancer survivors. However, sometimes therapists are intolerant of their own grieving and sense of loss. They may feel therapists should be strong and that grief at the death or illness of a client may reflect overinvolvement or countertransference. Of course, the nature and extent of the grieving should be assessed to determine whether it does reflect an unhealthy response. Therapists also should consider the possibility that their grief at the loss of a client may reflect a reactivation of their own earlier losses or reflect unwarranted guilt that they were not able to save the client. However, therapists need to realize that sadness over the death of a client is an understandable and natural reaction.

Therapists Who Are Also Cancer Survivors

Many therapists gravitate toward working with cancer survivors because of personal experience with cancer. Although I have been working with people with cancer for approximately fifteen years, my interest in this group intensified when close family members were diagnosed with cancer and when I too became a cancer survivor.

When cancer survivors are referred to me for treatment, usually they are aware that I have considerable experience in counseling cancer survivors and am a cancer survivor. If a cancer survivor comes to see me without this information or if a client I have been seeing for another reason presents issues related to cancer in themselves or a loved one, I volunteer the information that I am a cancer survivor but provide little information about my own experience unless they ask questions. I want to let them know I have a special understanding of their situation but do not want to take the attention away from their experience.

My own experience with cancer has both benefits and drawbacks in the therapeutic relationship. As one of my clients wrote, "It was extremely valuable having a nonjudgmental person who had gone through the same cancer ordeal listen to my rantings when others had turned me off. I also used my therapist as an inspiration." Knowing that I have had cancer and am doing well reassures my clients that people can survive the disease. It also gives me a special empathy and enables me to anticipate some of my clients' reactions to their disease and its treatments, to ask the right questions, and to take a preventive approach in helping them handle chemotherapy and other consequences of the disease.

Kane (1991) wrote of the "wounded healer": "Some of the most effective healers I know are people who have experienced chronic or major acute illnesses" (p. 109). Their own experience with life-threatening illness seems to deepen the understanding and capacity for insight of therapists who are also cancer survivors.

Another benefit of that experience is the bond it promotes between client and therapist. In the therapeutic setting, as well as in other arenas, rapport develops rapidly between people who are cancer survivors. Conversation quickly moves to an intimate level as people talk freely about their experience with cancer with someone who has been there. This rapid bonding between cancer survivors means that the therapeutic process seems to progress even more rapidly than usual, with little time spent on testing the relationship or trivial conversation. Understanding and acceptance seem to be assumed even before they are demonstrated and the development of rapport between therapist and client who are both cancer survivors is rarely difficult.

However, being a therapist who is a cancer survivor can also cause some difficulties. Clients frequently inquire about my experience, expecting that I will tell them exactly how it will be for them. Although I do share information about my own diagnosis and treatment with my clients if they request it, I limit the information I share, I emphasize that each person's reactions are different and theirs may be quite unlike mine, and I always allow time for them to explore what their experience has been. It is essential to keep the focus on the cancer survivor's experiences rather than my own. I also try to present more than one perspective, telling clients not only about my own experiences but also about those of people I have counseled or members of support groups I have worked with to help them see that the same treatment or experience may elicit very different reactions and that there is no one right way to react to or deal with cancer and its treatment.

Another drawback to being both therapist and cancer survivor is that some people are reluctant to share worries or bad news because they are afraid it might cause me to be upset or worried about my own health. In an effort to allay clients' fears, I introduce this issue early in the therapeutic relationship, before it becomes a concern, and let people know that this is a reaction they might have to receiving therapy from another cancer survivor. I assure them that I want to know all of their important thoughts, feelings, and experiences, even the negative ones. I let them know that of course if their treatments do not progress well or do not seem effective, I will feel saddened and concerned. However, sharing that experience is part of building a trusting and effective therapeutic relationship and I am ready to deal with any issues they want to raise.

Therapists with a history of cancer who relapse and have a poor prognosis may have particular difficulty providing psychotherapy to cancer survivors. The therapist's disease and deterioration will need to be addressed with the clients and, if the therapist is dying, efforts should be made to help clients deal with this and find another therapist.

In my own work, I saw several cancer survivors whose previous therapists had died of cancer. Not only did this present a great loss for the clients but it also escalated their own fears about the disease. They seemed to believe that if someone as capable and resourceful as their therapist could die of cancer, their own likelihood of surviving was not good. Other reactions to an activation of cancer in the therapist include concern, sadness and grief, anger, betrayal, withdrawal, protectiveness, resentment, and anticipation of abandonment (Flapan, 1986). These reactions may interfere with the therapeutic process.

At the same time, cancer in the therapist has also been found to have a beneficial impact on some clients. The therapist's illness can precipitate a breakthrough, since clients may believe their time with the therapist is limited and should be used productively (Flapan, 1986). Clients may also feel closer to the therapist and may be more willing to reveal their own fears and feelings of vulnerability. The therapist's illness also may prompt them to take better care of their health and may reduce any denial about the seriousness of the disease.

Overall, the benefits of therapists having had their own experience with cancer seem to far outweigh the risks. However, they do need to keep the possible pitfalls in mind and address them with their clients.

Overview of Chapter

This chapter has focused on the relationships between cancer survivors and their treatment providers, including both medical personnel and psychotherapists. Cancer affects these professional relationships just as it does relationships with family and friends, and psychotherapists should consider the impact of their clients' disease on themselves and on the clients' health care providers. By considering that impact, therapists can have a better understanding of their own reactions to their clients and can help them interact more successfully with the rest of their treatment team.

Helping People Cope with Recurrence, Death, and Loss

Despite the best efforts of the medical team, the support of family and friends, the fighting spirit of the cancer survivor, and the contributions of psychotherapy, many people will have one or more recurrences of cancer and some will die from the disease. Unfortunately, research on people with cancer has focused primarily on those in the first year of coping with an initial diagnosis and has not paid adequate attention to people with recurrent or advanced disease (Hopwood & Maguire, 1992). Available research as well as experience, however, does provide some information for therapists treating people with recurrences or advanced cancer. This chapter will look at the impact that recurrence has on cancer survivors and their families as well as ways to help people cope yet again with cancer. It will also discuss dying and death as well bereavement and mourning and ways therapists can help people dealing with severe losses.

Recurrence

For most cancer survivors, the initial diagnosis and treatment of cancer is followed by a period of apprehension and anxiety. The physical and psychological impact of the disease is still present, along with the fear of recurrence. Over months and years, this fear usually recedes, although few people report it disappears entirely.

Unfortunately, a symptom may lead to a test that may lead to the disappointing news that the disease has recurred. Particularly if the recurrence reflects a metastases or spread of the disease to another site, the prognosis may be worse than it was for the initial diagnosis. However, many people do survive recurrences and go on to lead lives free of cancer. A recurrence does not always mean that death is inevitable.

Emotional Reactions

Nevertheless, most cancer survivors react to a recurrence with initial pessimism, shock, and confusion (Simonton, Matthews-Simonton, & Creighton, 1992). Strong feelings of frustration, blame of oneself and one's medical treatment, disappointment, and hopelessness are common (Zimpfer, 1992). Concerns about the self, the impact of the disease on work and family, as well as existential concerns about the future and the meaning of life typically arise, as they do with an initial diagnosis of cancer.

Several differences between people's reactions to an initial diagnosis of cancer and their reactions to a recurrence are noteworthy:

Most people find they actually have more resources available to them than they did when they were dealing with the initial diagnosis (Sales, 1991). Coping mechanisms have been developed and relationships strengthened as a result of previous efforts to deal with cancer. People have more information and professional resources and now are dealing with familiar concepts and choices. Therapists can identify and reinforce successful coping strategies and can help people anticipate and avoid difficulties that arose the first time they had to deal with cancer.

However, feelings of self-blame, discouragement, anger, and hopelessness may be even stronger than they were with the initial diagnosis. Depression is more likely to be present after discovery of a first recurrence and during the terminal stage of the disease than after the initial diagnosis (Hughes, 1987). People may think, "I did everything possible to recover from cancer the first time and it didn't work; why should I bother trying again? There's no use." Family members too may blame themselves as well as the person with cancer, and this may contribute to discouragement and low self-esteem. These thoughts and feelings may prevent the person from actively pursuing treatment. Psychotherapy needs to determine whether these dysfunctional attitudes are present and if so to address them in therapy. Helping people explore the personal meaning they give to the recurrence as well as discussing their worst fears may bring these feelings to the surface and make them accessible to treatment.

Extreme reactions of denial or hopelessness may also prevent people from making decisions that will be needed if they do not recover. People may fear that talking about death will make it happen and may avoid any discussion that is not positive. Therapists can address this denial gently by suggesting an attitude of "hope for the best but prepare for the worst." Hatfield and Hatfield (1992) described this as "what if " thinking, a willingness to consider and prepare for all options and possibilities. If people can adopt this attitude, they then can be encouraged to take such steps as making wills and visiting places they have always longed to see, without fearing it will hasten their deaths.

However, extreme pessimism may lead people to withdraw from life. One woman with a recurrence of breast cancer believed her death was inevitable and sought to prepare for that by reading books about death and dying, planning her funeral, and visualizing herself wasting away. Rather than easing her fears, this increased her depression and alienated people in her support systems who were struggling to maintain a hopeful attitude. Here, too, a realistic optimism that considers the possibility of survival as well as of death seems most effective in promoting emotional adjustment and appropriate action.

Helping People Cope with Recurrences

In most respects, psychotherapy with people who have a recurrence of cancer is similar to therapy for people with an initial diagnosis of cancer. Most of the guidelines and suggestions made earlier in this book are pertinent here too.

Therapists need to view cancer survivors in context and gather information about their support systems, their views of illness and medical treatments, and their lifestyles. Obtaining medical information on treatment options, likely repercussions of treatment, and the prognosis of the disease is important. Essential to treatment planning is information on how people coped with cancer initially: what coping skills they used, how effective those skills were, what support systems were available, what strengths and choices helped people deal with the disease, and what obstacles they encountered in their fight against cancer.

Cognitive-behavioral techniques can help people cope with their anxiety and depression, build up their sense of self-efficacy, and make sound decisions. Existential and affective interventions can provide reassurance, support, and a sense of meaning to people's lives. Family and group counseling can promote support, effective communication, and the development of positive interpersonal relationships.

In addition, interventions that enable people to deal with the possibility of death are even more important than they were during the initial diagnosis of cancer. These interventions are discussed in detail in the next section of this chapter and include ways to help people appreciate the meaning of their lives, take practical steps to plan for the possibility of death, leave a legacy, resolve any conflicts or unfinished business with family or friends, and maintain hope and control as much and as long as possible. People who are close to the person with a recurrence will also need help in managing their own feelings, in getting the support and help they need, and in providing practical and emotional support to the person with cancer.

Helping Family Members Cope

Family members too may react with even more depression and anxiety than they did to the initial diagnosis of cancer. Especially if the

recurrence is diagnosed within the first year or so of the initial diagnosis, family resources may be depleted. Family members may feel
emotionally drained, have already used up their savings to pay for
treatment of the initial disease, and may feel reluctant to ask others for more help with child care and meal preparation. Time away
from work already may have interfered with job performance. People may think that they cannot possibly cope with cancer again.
Anger at the medical team, as well as at the person with cancer,
may also make it difficult for them to move forward with plans to
deal with the recurrence.

Coping with these strong reactions may be especially difficult
because people usually do not want to contribute further to the
stress and upset of the person with cancer. Consequently, family
members who are very concerned and involved may appear to withdraw and withhold communication. This may be misinterpreted by
the person with cancer as rejection or disinterest, leading to tension and conflict in relationships. This misunderstanding can compound the already difficult task of coping with the recurrence.

Families with considerable dysfunction as well as families with
extreme and rigid beliefs are likely to have particular difficulty dealing with a recurrence (Rolland, 1994). They may hold firmly to a
belief that willpower or prayer can cure cancer and may have trouble recognizing that even those powerful forces may not be able to
overcome bad fortune. Families may pressure themselves to expend
increasing efforts to combat the disease, may seek out alternate and
questionable treatments, and may seem unable to accept a poor
prognosis. As a result, the family as well as the person with cancer
may fail to make good use of the time they have left, may not
resolve relationships and make appropriate financial and medical
decisions, and may approach death with denial and self-blame.

Helping family members to share their reactions to the recurrence, to explore their fears, to develop realistic hopes and plans,
and to make sound decisions are the tasks of the psychotherapist.
Achieving these goals through individual and family therapy can
make an important difference in the emotional and physical health

of the person with cancer and the life of the family, whatever the outcome of the recurrence.

Dying and Death

Approximately five hundred thousand people die from cancer each year (McDaniel, Hepworth, & Doherty, 1992). Few studies are available on the emotional and physical process of dying from cancer, presumably because collecting data from people going through that experience is viewed as both difficult and intrusive. However, those studies that are available, as well as the general literature on dying and death, provide useful information for psychotherapists working with people with cancer who are terminally ill.

Characteristics of the Terminally Ill Person

Doka (1993) described the terminal phase of an illness, the time when the chance of recovery or remission is remote, as the time when the goal changes from curing or maintaining remission to providing palliative care. Most people sense when their death is imminent, although both physical and emotional reactions differ considerably among people in the terminal stage of cancer (Moorey & Greer, 1989). According to Selfridge (1990), "the terminal cancer patient experiences denial, pent-up anger, guilt, helplessness, being out of control, curtailment of the future, goals left unattained, hopes abandoned, and threats to self-esteem through an increasing dependence . . . " (p. 192). High anxiety is, not surprisingly, common during this period but depression seems to be even more common (Payne, 1989). At the same time, neither emotion is found in some people with advanced cancer. Self-absorption is another common reaction of people who are dying (Doka, 1993).

No consistent correlation has been found between the severity of the disease and either self-esteem or psychological adjustment. According to Doka (1993, p. 1), "Each of us will die much as we live. . . . Thus it is useful to explore the ways one has responded to crisis in the past. Often we can be expected to show similar reactions now."

Four typical orientations to death have been observed:

1. *Constructive coping:* Acceptance, transcendence, defiance
2. *Indirect coping:* Bargaining, postponing, experimenting with unproven treatments, prayer
3. *Avoidance:* Denial, disdain, repression
4. *Discouragement:* Hopelessness, hastening death, fearfulness, capitulation

While constructive coping may be viewed as the ideal way to meet death, the other orientations also have a place in the process of helping people to prepare themselves for death and may represent steps toward constructive coping. People with strong religious beliefs as well as those without religious beliefs seem to fare better than those with confused beliefs. Having successful experiences negotiating past crises can also help people deal with the crisis of dying. However, almost everyone can benefit from help in dealing with this very difficult final crisis and most people need and want to talk about their situation (Doka, 1993).

Psychotherapy During the Terminal Stage of Cancer

Psychotherapy has a great deal to offer people with cancer, even in the final weeks or months of their lives. Therapy for people with advanced cancer has been found to reduce stress and depression, improve self-esteem and satisfaction with life, promote a greater sense of control, improve relationships, and reduce pain and fear of death (Andersen, 1992; Linn, Linn, & Harris, 1982). Treatment during this period should usually include the following:

Empathy. In itself, empathy is therapeutic. It can provide comfort and support and helps reduce the isolation and withdrawal that often accompanies the final stage of cancer.

Opportunity to express and explore feelings. People who are dying usually have many strong feelings, including worry, fear, depression, anger, guilt, helplessness, disappointment, and blame. Identifying and sorting out these feelings can help them see that the feelings are manageable and that in fact some of those feelings can be alleviated. It also can help them face the apparent inevitability of their deaths.

For example, fear of death typically includes apprehension about the process of dying, worry about pain and suffering, concern about the consequences the death will have for loved ones, existential fear of death itself, and concern about the afterlife. Kübler-Ross (1981) found that many people described these feelings as a "fear of a catastrophic destructive force bearing down" (p. 20). Asking questions such as, "What are you feeling? What do you think is happening?" may help people to talk about their fears. Drawing or other expressive approaches to dealing with feelings also may be helpful, especially for children who are facing death.

Some people with advanced cancer may isolate themselves in preparation for their deaths. They may even long for death to end a difficult and painful process. These feelings too should be accepted and understood, although therapists usually will also seek to help people maximize their involvement and activities.

Help in obtaining information to allay fears. Helping people communicate and ask questions of their physicians may help allay fears about the process of dying. Physicians usually can assure people that medications are available that are effective in reducing pain associated with the final stages of cancer and that these will be provided as needed. Physicians can also reassure people that these medications almost never cause psychological addiction, another common fear of people in the terminal phase of cancer (Farrow, Cash, & Simmons, 1990). Talking with family members and making sure the family will be provided for can reduce concern about the impact of the death on others. Even the existential fear of death can be reduced through discussion of beliefs and using therapy to make sense and meaning of one's life.

A variety of psychotherapeutic interventions. Affective as well as cognitive and behavioral techniques can be used to elicit automatic thoughts, promote expression of feeling, and help people discuss and cope with their impending death. Many of the interventions discussed in Chapters Five and Six of this book are useful during the final stages of cancer. In addition, some techniques have been described in the literature that are designed especially for use during this stage.

Previous experiences with dying and death are likely to color the present experience and may serve as a focus for initiating difficult discussions. Therapists should not pressure people to confront this topic but rather should let clients be the guide, with the therapist providing a safe and accepting presence that will promote self-disclosure. Techniques such as visualization and relaxation can help people summon up their visions of what dying and death will be like for them and reduce the fear associated with those stages. If feelings threaten to become overwhelming or incapacitating, techniques such as distraction or positive avoidance may restore self-control.

Simonton, Matthews-Simonton, and Creighton (1992) promoted awareness of feelings about dying and death by encouraging people with advanced cancer to visualize themselves moving toward death, dying, and then experiencing the aftermath of death. They then imagined returning to life and creating a plan for the rest of their lives. A similar process also has been used with friends and family to help them confront fears of losing a loved one and of the unknown (Combs, 1992). This experience apparently is not as difficult as most people expect it will be and can improve the quality of both living and dying. However, a death fantasy should be used with great care, and generally should be reserved for people with good ego strength and personal resources.

Smith, Richards, and Maher (1993) suggested other creative approaches to help people who are terminally ill. The following techniques all involve changing the dying person's images or metaphors into ones that are more positive and comforting:

Empty chair: A role play in which the dying person has a dialogue with cancer, death, pain, or any other important concept or feeling or with an important person with whom the survivor has unfinished business.

Reducing pain through metaphor and imagery: Physical sensations are visualized and modified. For example, a person may imagine pain flowing into the hands and then being discarded.

Relaxation and guided imagery: Developing affirmations and images based on the metaphors the person has of the dying process can be used to enable them to visualize death as a place of peace and comfort.

Energy transformation: Negative energy such as worry or pain is transformed into positive activities such as listing special moments in one's life.

Facilitating sound decision making. People dealing with terminal cancer, as well as their families and close friends, have many decisions to make including decisions about treatment, care of the person with cancer, management of other family responsibilities, wills, and funeral arrangements. Therapists can promote communication between people with cancer and their loved ones to help them consider their choices and make the best decisions they can. Maximizing the involvement of people with cancer in this process can give them a sense of control and help them feel that they continue to play an important and respected part in the family. It also can reassure them that all efforts will be made to ensure that they will not suffer and will have the sort of death they want. The process of making decisions can be facilitated if therapists also help people obtain the information they need from physicians, insurance companies, financial advisers, and others and familiarize them with resources such as hospices that can help them deal with the process of dying and death.

Maximizing quality of life. Helping people identify what they still can and want to accomplish in their lives and enabling them to achieve those goals may imbue even their last days with a sense of purpose, control, and accomplishment. Rawnsley (1990) suggested asking, "How can we help you to live as fully as possible under the conditions imposed by cancer and its treatment?" (p. 205). Finding an answer to this question can help people with terminal cancer realize that they are still alive and can separate death from their present reality. Realistic goals should be established, perhaps focused on the practical steps needed to prepare for death or on communicating feelings to friends and family. Even small steps such as making a telephone call or asking someone to obtain information on a living will can give a sense of achievement. Scheduling realistic daily activities can also help reduce depression and anxiety and fill up time that might otherwise be devoted to worry and ruminating. Something as simple as a plan to watch a video or spend time with a friend can give the person with cancer something to anticipate and can improve mood and energy level.

Establishing goals and maintaining a sense of direction are also important in instilling hope. While unrealistic optimism is usually not desirable because it can prevent people from taking necessary steps to prepare for their death, realistic hope has a place for people who are dying. Hope can give them a sense that life is worth living and a reason to go on, even in the final stages of the disease. Realistic hopes might include leaving one's family well taken care of and prepared for the death and feeling peaceful and pain-free for the remainder of one's life. In addition, many cases have been reported of people who had been diagnosed with terminal cancer but whose disease went into remission for many years. The possibility of such a recovery should not be completely discounted, although it should not be expected.

Helping people make meaning of their lives. Some of the existential fears of people who are dying have to do with a concern that their lives have not been meaningful and that they will be forgotten when they die. LeShan (1989) observed that the process of dying can add meaning to life and can be a time of growth and self-acceptance. Therapists who give people the opportunity to tell their life stories, to share photographs and other mementos, to listen to favorite songs, to identify and congratulate themselves on their successes and accomplishments, can help them feel a sense of purpose and wholeness about their lives. Discussion focused on such topics as lessons learned from life, best and worst experiences, regrets, and what I need to do to forgive myself and others not only will give a sense of meaning to a person's life but can pave the way for healing relationships and leaving a legacy.

People who are dying often feel a need for integration, a return to their origins, either in their mind or in reality (LeShan, 1989). A life review also can help people achieve that sense of integration, an understanding of why their life evolved as it did.

Some people derive a sense of meaning and comfort from their religious and philosophical beliefs. Finding a way to leave a legacy that reflects their values can also add a sense of meaning and continuity to people's lives. Gilda Radner, the well-known comedian who died of ovarian cancer, did this by writing a book about her experiences with cancer; by initiating the establishment of Gilda's Club, a facility in New York providing support and help to people with cancer; and by developing a data bank designed to assist people in identifying whether they have a family history of some cancers. Although few people can have such a profound impact, therapists can help people identify a way they can leave a meaningful legacy. Parents with young children have written letters, compiled photograph albums, or made audio- or videotapes to be shared with their children. One man dictated the history of his family and had it transcribed and distributed to all his relatives. Another man who had been an artist established a scholarship in his name at a local college to help needy students purchase art supplies. Dying with strength, dignity, and caring, setting a model that will help others in their grief and with their own lives, is yet another kind of legacy.

Making arrangements for the death. Family members, as well as people who are dying, can gain great peace of mind from making practical arrangements that will facilitate decision making as death approaches. The Patient Self-Determination Act of 1991 requires medical facilities to inform people of their right to refuse treatment or have life supports turned off (Winograd, 1992). This mandates that people's advanced directives will be honored. A living will can reassure people with cancer that only those medical interventions they request will be performed. Some people may prefer that all medical procedures be done to prolong their lives while others specify that ventilators, feeding tubes, and cardiopulmonary resuscitation not be used but that only pain medication and fluids be provided toward the end. Establishment of a durable power of attorney, specifying who can make decisions if the ill person is incapacitated, can also assure people that their wishes will be carried out.

Traditional wills specifying distribution of assets and possessions are also needed and can reassure people with cancer as well as their loved ones that their wishes will be carried out. Leaving special bequests such as jewelry or books to family or friends is another way to leave a meaningful legacy, reminding others of close bonds and relationships. Family members should be informed of the location of important papers and provided with information on life insurance, social security, and other resources that will be essential to them.

Finally, plans need to be made for the funeral and burial or cremation. For many, this will be the most difficult effort, bringing home the reality that the person is dying. However, if possible, people who are approaching death should be given the opportunity to express their preferences so that the details of the funeral are not made hastily and under great stress after the death has occurred. In addition, the rituals associated with the death are most likely to be meaningful and comforting if they reflect the style and preferences of the family and the person who has died.

Resolving relationships, receiving support, and saying goodbye. For the dying and those close to them, resolving conflicts in relationships, expressing mutual love and appreciation, dealing with feelings of separation and loss, and finally saying goodbye are important as well as difficult aspects of the process of dying. Therapists should review with clients who their important relationships are, what problems or unfinished concerns remain in those relationships, and what can be done to restore closeness. Therapists can help people to plan ways to communicate with their family and friends and may want to be present to facilitate that process. Promoting communication between the dying person and significant others can also increase the support the person receives and maintain a sense of self-worth. Being able to talk explicitly about the approaching death generally increases closeness and eases both the dying process and the grief of loved ones (Sales, Schultz, & Biegel, 1992). Touch as well as words seem especially important to communicate caring in a person's last weeks (Farrow, Cash, & Simmons, 1990).

Family and friends should be encouraged to talk with the dying person, continuing to express love and appreciation, telling the person what a good life he or she has lived and how he or she will be remembered, until the person has died. Hearing is the last sense to deteriorate even in a comatose state, and messages of caring and praise can help the dying person as well as those who are expressing their feelings (Rolland, 1994).

Group Psychotherapy

Group counseling, as well as individual and family counseling, can be as helpful to people with terminal cancer as to people in the initial stages of cancer. Selfridge (1990) formed therapy groups of people who had an estimated survival time of three to six months and who did not have adequate external support systems. Groups consisted of five to seven members and met for six weekly sessions. Members had a great deal to contribute to each other and benefited from the sharing as well as from the establishment of cohesive and trusting relationships. Group members provided support, promoted development of coping skills, reduced loneliness and isolation, ameliorated anxiety, mobilized trust, provided an opportunity for self-expression, and contributed to each other's self-esteem. Members were fearful of each other's deaths and sometimes the healthier members avoided those who were sicker than they were, while the very ill tended to withdraw. Nevertheless, the mutual grieving helped people in the groups to cope with the loss of members. The benefits of the groups seemed to outweigh any difficulties that arose.

Baron (1985) too suggested support groups for people who are terminally ill and conceptualized those groups as being for the living, not the dying. Baron's groups not only provided support but also helped participants deal with everyday problems that arose.

Spiegel viewed support groups as a way to help people with both the physical and emotional aspects of late-stage disease (Moyers, 1993). According to Spiegel, "If you can't control whether or not you die, you can at least control how you live and how your body is handling the stressors that you're facing" (p. 158). He found that self-hypnosis helped people to manage pain while group support and a focus on common experiences and emotions assisted people in dealing with fear and depression. Mourning of members who died was reassuring rather than discouraging and helped people appreciate their own importance.

The Process of Dying

In her work with people who were dying, Kübler-Ross (1981) identified five stages in the dying process: (1) denial and isolation ("no, not me"), (2) anger and bargaining, (3) preparatory grief (mourning the death and future losses), (4) resignation (defeat and bitterness), and (5) acceptance (a sense of victory, peace and serenity, submitting to things we cannot change). Similar stages may be observed in family members who are going through anticipatory grief.

These stages are not necessarily sequential; people may move back and forth from one stage to another. In addition, many people do not experience all five stages. However, Kübler-Ross's model provides a useful framework for looking at the process of dying. By comparing a person's own responses to dying with this model, therapists can obtain a better understanding of what feelings have surfaced, the process the person is going through in an effort to come to terms with impending death, what barriers that person may be encountering, and how therapy can help the person to reach acceptance.

Therapists should assess how family members as well as the person with cancer are coping with the process of dying. Tension and communication difficulties may develop when family members and the dying person are at different stages of Kübler-Ross's model.

Death resulting from cancer is usually a gradual process. Feelings of profound fatigue may indicate that death is approaching (LeShan, 1989). The person increasingly weakens, withdraws, and may stop eating and drinking. Periods of unconsciousness may increase, sometimes leading to a comatose state (Barraclough, 1994). Cognitive impairment is common in people with advanced or terminal cancer (Hughes, 1987). Helping people with cancer as well as their friends and families to anticipate this process can provide some reassurance and can reduce upset at the hallmarks of the dying process.

The Impact of Dying and Death on Family and Friends

According to Kübler-Ross (1981, p. 47), "If the family can finish their unfinished business before a patient dies, then there is no grief work to do whatsoever after death, although there will always be the natural grief." Families (defined here as both biological family and intimates) struggle to deal with the loss of a loved one, both before and after the death. By understanding the process of anticipatory grieving as well as common ways of responding to bereavement, therapists can better help families to grieve in a positive and comforting way. Without help, family members seem more likely to experience unresolved or conflicted grief, which can take an emotional and physical toll on the bereaved. Husbands of women who died of breast cancer, for example, showed suppressed immune functioning for the first year after the death (Redd & Jacobson, 1988).

How people react to a bereavement is determined by many factors including past experiences in dealing with loss, their emotional style and coping skills, the role of the deceased and their relationship with that person, the duration and nature of the illness, and coexisting stressors. Families typically have implicit guidelines that determine how they should react to a bereavement; helping people become aware of these family messages may help them become more aware of their own feelings. In addition, putting the grief in context can help both therapists and the people who are grieving understand their reactions.

Common reactions to a bereavement include denial; anger at oneself, at the person with cancer, and at the physicians; anguish; guilt; anxiety about decisions; confusion; numbing; sadness; vulnerability; and relief. Feelings of role overload, isolation, exhaustion, and inadequacy are also common, especially for family members who are caring at home for the person with cancer (Sales, 1991). Some feelings such as anger at the dying person and guilt at feeling relieved to be free of caretaking responsibilities may be troubling to people, although they are common and understandable.

Family members may also worry about their own futures and ability to cope. As one wife wrote, "My identity came from him, and if you don't have a sense of identity beyond the other person, the death is devastating." Old family issues may be reactivated, and some family members may cope with their stress through bickering and recriminations. Other family members suppress their feelings to avoid saddening those around them or out of discomfort with their own strong emotions. One caretaker said, "I kept thinking, if he can cope and he is dying, who am I to complain? If he can deal with it, so can I." Acting out and physical symptoms can also be manifestations of grief.

While some people feel anticipatory grief, others will not really experience their grief until months after the death. However, most seem to have some kind of strong emotional reaction when the death occurs. People may have a vivid sense of seeing, hearing, or feeling the presence of the deceased. The aftermath of the death is also a time when shock, disorganization, and anxiety may increase; before that, people may have been protected by the structure of their caretaking roles. When those roles are gone, disorientation may set in.

Stages of Grieving

For most people, the individual grieving process involves a series of steps (Doka, 1993):

1.   *Accepting the reality of the loss.* Talking about the loss with others and expressing one's own feelings is usually the first step. Rituals such as funerals, wakes, and sitting shivah can facilitate this process. Therapists can use questioning to help people review the dying process and actualize it.

2.   *Facing one's grief.* People need to become aware of and express their reactions to the loss, to work through the pain and grief, and to deal with any guilt and unfinished business.

3.   *Adjusting to life without the person.* Many people need at least six months to reorient themselves to life without the person who has died and to relinquish their old attachments and assumptions. This process seems to be most successful if it is a gradual process rather than a flight from loneliness into rapid and extreme changes and involvements.

4.   *Finding ways to remember the person who has died.* Family members need to ensure that their loved one will be remembered. They may initiate rituals to mark the death—lighting memorial candles on the anniversary of the death or gathering at the gravesite on special dates. Rituals such as these promote healing. Therapists should help people develop mourning rituals that are consistent

with their cultural and religious background as well as with their feelings toward the deceased.

Many ways are available to remember and honor the person who has died. Contributions to the American Cancer Society or other organizations with particular meaning to the family can be made in memory of the deceased. Poems and tributes can be written about the person who has died or letters can be composed to be read at the gravesite. If resources permit, scholarships may be established, trees may be planted, or other concrete reminders may be cotab- lished in memory of the person. Children as well as adults may ben- efit from developing a memory book with photographs, drawings, and writing about the person. Journal keeping, visits to former fam- ily homes and the deceased's birthplace, and talking with people who knew the person are other ways to honor and remember the deceased.

5. *Rebuilding faith and belief systems*. Religious and spiritual beliefs and practices can be a great comfort to people who have experienced a bereavement. At the same time, the death, particu- larly if it was painful and early in the person's life, may have seemed unfair and may have raised religious doubts and questions. These doubts may need to be addressed and beliefs reassessed as a result of a death.

6. *Developing a changed identity and reconstructing one's life*. If the person who died was central to the life of the bereaved, life as it had been may need to be much changed. People need to find ways to move on with their lives without forgetting what they have left behind. Worden (1991) described this as emotionally relocating the deceased and going forward with life. New goals and relationships may need to be formed, not as replacements for the old ones but as other ways to give meaning and direction to life. Energy can then be gradually redirected from involvement with the deceased to involvement with new activities and relationships.

Families go through steps in their grief as do individuals. Rosen (1990) delineated four steps as important to grieving as a family:

(1) shared acknowledgment of the reality of death, (2) shared experience of the pain of grief, (3) reorganization of the family roles and system in light of the loss of an important family member, and (4) redirection and reinvestment of the family's energy, relationships, and goals. Accomplishment of these four steps takes most families at least a year (Rosen, 1990). Anticipatory grief, as well as mourning after a death, are usually most comforting and healing when they are interactive and supportive processes involving the family system. Use of genograms and family stories can facilitate grieving and help link the present loss to the family history of loss and bereavement, making it more meaningful by putting it in context.

Although the severity of grief diminishes over time for most people, it is usually not a smooth process and its course and duration cannot be predicted. People typically experience grief in waves, triggered by thoughts, memories, or experiences that recall the deceased. Renewed feelings of grief at special dates such as the anniversary of the death or the birthday of the person who died are common. Another frequent pattern is intensification of grief in the third year after the death (Pine & Brauer, 1986).

Problematic Grief Reactions

Many signs of abnormal grief have been identified including viewing the deceased in extreme terms (perfect or terrible), confusion or disagreement about the treatment and cause of death, endless discussion or no discussion of the deceased, unexplained and prolonged anger and resentment toward the person who died, strong feelings of guilt, exaggerated and disabling grief, inhibited or absent grief, assumption of traits of the deceased, grief that manifests itself through physical or emotional symptoms that are attributed to other causes, severe depression and suicidal ideation, very delayed mourning, and interminable mourning and yearning for the deceased (Chochinov, 1993; Rosen, 1990; Vachon, 1987). Bowen (1991) wrote of aftershocks following a death, disruptions in the overall family functioning such as illnesses, substance use, or problems at school or work.

Helping Family Members with Anticipatory Grief

Family members, like people in the terminal stage of cancer, need to take an active role in the dying process, for themselves as well as for their loved one. They can express appreciation for the dying person and promote a sense of accomplishment in that person. Talking, touching, and just being with the person with cancer can be mutually comforting, whether or not the person seems to hear or understand. Caretaking tasks, even for someone who is in the hospital, can be reassuring and help people feel they are making a contribution. Family members need to participate in discussions of advanced directives and funeral arrangements so that they know the wishes of the dying person and are sure they are fulfilling them later.

Family members, like people who are dying, need to explore their own images of death. They also are likely to benefit from imagining how their lives will be different without the bereaved and developing plans to cope with that loss.

Some families participate in a sort of deathwatch, in which family members alternate being with the dying person until death comes. This can be both emotionally and physically draining. Family members should not be dissuaded from this if they believe it is important; being present at the time of death and having time with the deceased immediately after death has been found to help people accept the reality of the death and deal with the loss more successfully (Chochinov, 1993). However, family members may need help in setting realistic demands for themselves and processing their strong feelings. If the deathwatch is a prolonged one, family members may also need help in retaining some of the normal aspects of life and attending to the needs of children and other family members who may be neglected.

People with cancer sometimes need permission to die (Doka, 1993). They may fight an inevitable death out of fear of abandoning or letting down the family, causing themselves pain and discomfort. If this seems to be the case, therapists may raise the possibility of the family giving the person with cancer permission to die. This can be a statement that is repeated such as, "You've had a wonderful life. You've accomplished a great deal. We all love you very much. You've fought a long fight against cancer, but it's all right to let go now. We know you have done your best."

Helping People Mourn

As Farrow, Cash, and Simmons (1990, p. 15) wrote, "Witnessing the death of a loved one is one of the most difficult tasks anyone can face." Therapists can do a great deal to ease this process. Worden (1991) identified ten ways in which counseling can help people work through grief:

1. Help actualize the loss
2. Help people to identify and express feelings
3. Help them go on with life without the deceased
4. Facilitate withdrawal of emotions from the deceased
5. Provide time and a place to grieve
6. Normalize reactions
7. Allow for individual differences
8. Provide continuous support
9. Help people to manage defenses and develop coping skills
10. Treat abnormal reactions or psychopathology

Helping people mourn begins with helping them express and absorb their feelings. The process of venting feelings can bring a sense of relief and hope of feeling better, especially if therapists help people recognize that their reactions are normal and understandable. Discussion of the death, family genograms that highlight past losses, and films and books on loss and death all can help people become aware of their feelings and express them to the therapist as well as to other family members. Reviewing family roles and responsibilities, the place the deceased held in the family, and religious and culturally based conceptions of families, illness, and death can provide further information on the mourning process. The current bereavement may bring back memories of prior losses that will affect the mourning process and may need attention. People who had dependent, ambivalent, or conflicted relationships with the person who died are particularly likely to have difficulty with the mourning process (Vachon, 1987).

Relationships and Mourning

The nature of the relationship a person has had with the deceased is likely to have a profound impact on the mourning process. Therapists should consider both the quality and the nature of the relationship when assessing grief reactions.

Mourning the Death of a Child

Parents whose children die commonly have great difficulty accepting that loss; it seems unjust and unbelievable. The whole meaning of their lives is threatened. As one parent said after the death of her son, "I just lost a lot of my life. I couldn't tolerate seeing kids, having people talk about their kids." Losing a child involves not only the loss of a loved one but the loss of possibilities, grandchildren, the child's career success, and help in the parents' old age. Role redefinition and reinvesting are especially difficult for bereaved parents as is expression of their grief; they may feel they need to be strong for the rest of the family (Rando, 1986b, 1986c).

Extreme grief is common in parents who lose adult children as well as those who lose young children. Grief in parents of adult children may be particularly difficult because others may not expect them to grieve; attention may focus on the spouse and children, while parents may find themselves with only limited information and involvement in the death of their child (Rando, 1986a).

Therapists may need to normalize the parents' grief and help them seek the support and knowledge they need to deal with their child's death.

Parents whose child has died are particularly prone to guilt reactions. Miles and Demi (1986) described six types of guilt that often have been found in bereaved parents: (1) survivor guilt, (2) guilt regarding decisions and actions that affected the child's prognosis, (3) guilt about real or imagined problems in the relationship, (4) guilt related to moral or religious beliefs about punishment and justice, (5) guilt related to role performance, and (6) guilt about how grief is being expressed. These feelings may be very difficult for parents to acknowledge and discuss. Therapists can help people to anticipate and accept these feelings so that they can work them through.

Death of a child can be devastating to marriages. Inhibition of sexual response is a common consequence of such a loss (Rando, 1986b). Divorce rates as high as 80 percent have been reported for bereaved parents (McGoldrick & Walsh, 1991). Parenting also may be adversely affected since parents often overprotect and focus on their remaining children.

The Impact of Bereavement on Children and Adolescents

Adolescents or children who experience a bereavement, a loss of either a parent or a sibling, sometimes have difficulty grieving overtly. They may want to appear strong to their peers and family. However, by concealing their feelings, they may experience an additional loss through withdrawal from their family or their family's withdrawal from them. Children who have experienced a bereavement often become fearful of losing other loved ones and being left alone in an unsafe world. These common fears and responses can lead to prolonged grief reactions in children as well as physical complaints and acting-out behavior. Other common responses that children have to bereavement include anger at the family members who may be idealizing or focusing on the person who died, a wish that they themselves had died instead, an intense desire to return to normal, feeling cheated, fearing closeness, and experiencing discomfort with the mourning process, in addition to many other feelings that are common to all people experiencing a bereavement (Call, 1990).

Support, discussion, books, and films can reassure children, provide information, normalize their feelings, and promote expression of grief reactions. Peer groups in which children have the opportunity to share feelings with others who have experienced a bereavement have also been found to be helpful (Call, 1990).

Young Adults' Loss of a Parent

Young adults who lose a parents typically have particular difficulty mourning. They may feel torn between their family of origin and their new lives and may minimize the impact the loss has had on them (McGoldrick & Walsh, 1991). They may rush into establishment of their own families following the parent's death or, especially if they are the oldest, may have difficulty separating from their family of origin.

Death of a Spouse

Loss of a spouse is difficult at any age; 20 percent of people who have been widowed manifest an emotional disorder, usually depression, in the year after the bereavement (Barraclough, 1994). For many bereaved spouses, grief is compounded by feeling exhausted and depleted by months of caregiving. Death of a spouse seems particularly difficult for people who have not yet started a family or who have young children. They have lost not only a companion and helper but also their dreams of a shared future. In addition, their friends may be frightened by their experience and may fail to give them the support they need. Older people who are widowed are at especially high risk of death and suicide themselves during the first year after the bereavement, especially if they have had little time for anticipatory grieving.

Importance of Support for the Bereaved

Encouraging people to mobilize and make good use of their support systems can help them deal with the loss and grieving they are experiencing. Clergy, friends, other family members, colleagues, and of course the therapist are important sources of support. In addition, family members who are absorbed with their own grief may need help in providing support to each other and recognizing that can ease the pain of both the giver and the receiver of the support.

Support groups can help people of all ages to mourn and heal after a death. These may be natural support groups, comprised of family and friends, or groups offered through hospices or other programs to help the bereaved. The Candlelighters Childhood Cancer Foundation (see Resources), for example, is an organization that offers peer support for parents who have lost a child to cancer as well as for the child's siblings. Grieving with others can normalize reactions, build bonds, and strengthen families. As a mother who lost a child to cancer said, "There is nothing you can say when an innocent child dies in great pain, fully aware. But I needed to have friends with whom I could let my hair down and laugh."

Therapists' Own Feelings About Death

Psychotherapy with people who have experienced a bereavement may be difficult for therapists, especially if they had treated the person with cancer and are feeling their own loss at the death. Focusing on bereavement in psychotherapy may raise the therapist's own unresolved feelings of grief and loss and well as fears of losses that might be.

Particularly if the therapist knew the deceased, some sharing of one's own feelings is appropriate as long as it does not shift the focus away from the clients' feelings. Becoming tearful and sad when losses are described also is acceptable. Being with people who have suffered a loss can be very reassuring.

Of course, therapists should refrain from judging reactions, providing false reassurance, or predicting how people will feel. At the same time, describing typical reactions to bereavement, including a gradual recovery over time, can be reassuring and can help people view their responses as understandable and manageable.

Despite the pain and sadness therapists typically will feel at the death of a client, psychotherapy with dying people and their families can be very rewarding. Helping people cope with feelings they may only be able to discuss with the therapist, seeing that therapy can make a difference even in the process of dying, and continuing to help the family recover after the death can be a meaningful and enriching experience for therapists, can develop new skills and enhance the old ones, and can help them deal more successfully with their own feelings of loss. Therapists can take pride in their willingness and ability to address such painful issues with their clients and may develop a deeper appreciation of their own lives and those of their clients through helping families deal with death.

For therapists, as well as for people with cancer and their families, dealing with recurrences, deaths, and losses can be extremely painful and difficult. However, it also can be very rewarding to find that psychotherapy can help people cope even with the final stages of cancer.

Overview of Chapter

This chapter has focused on recurrence, dying, and death. Even in the final stages of cancer, therapists have a great deal to offer people who are terminally ill and their friends and family. Helping them cope with loss and grief, understand the dying process, mobilize their support systems, and bring a rewarding close to relationships can make a difference for the dying person as well as the bereaved friends and family members.

12

. . . .

Life as a Cancer Survivor

Long-term cancer survivors are a large and growing segment of the population. In the 1930s, fewer than 20 percent of people who had been diagnosed with cancer were alive five years later. Now, 50 percent will live at least five years. More than six million Americans or 2 percent of the population are cancer survivors (Mullan & Hoffman, 1990). Cancer survivors now have their own organization, the National Coalition for Cancer Survivorship, founded in 1986 (see Resources).

Changes After Cancer

Simonton, Matthews-Simonton, and Creighton (1992, p. 77) wrote of the cancer survivor, "The recovered patient is weller than well." Mullan and Hoffman (1990, p. 1) wrote, "No matter how troubling the symptoms and the treatments, survival from day to day, week to week, and year to year constitutes an enormous personal and human triumph over what might have been." People who cope with cancer and survive seem to develop new strengths and perspectives. As mentioned earlier, the Chinese pictogram for crisis combines the signs for danger and opportunity (Borysenko, 1988). Similarly, the word *crisis* is derived from the Greek word *krisis*, which means "decision" or "turning point." People who successfully pass through the crisis phase of cancer have faced danger and decisions but also have the opportunity for change and growth.

For most, many of these changes are beneficial. As one cancer survivor wrote, "Many positive things have come as a result of my cancer diagnosis: my new faith in God, a better understanding of myself, and a closer relationship with my husband and children. I feel that I wasn't truly adult until I had cancer. I discovered that I could face everyone's worst fear and survive."

For others, however, the loss is great: "Cutting out the cancer left emotional scars that were so much worse than the physical ones and would take so much longer to heal. I no longer have an unthreatened sense of future; there are now no long-term plans. If you no longer have dreams, you no longer have life. I feel I have already lost a great deal of life to cancer." Clearly, cancer survivors have powerful and mixed reactions in the aftermath of their disease and its treatment.

Stages of Cancer

Cancer can be thought of as a disease with three possible phases: crisis, chronic, and terminal. The *crisis stage* of the initial diagnosis and subsequent treatment has been discussed earlier in this book. Following the crisis stage, most people enter the *chronic phase* in which there is both hope that the person has been cured and fear that the disease might recur. The term *chronic* is used to describe this period because cancer survivors must continue to cope with the physical and psychological aftermath of the disease and generally will not be viewed as cured for many years. For some, the chronic phase is brief, perhaps lasting only a few months before a recurrence or metastasis of the disease is discovered. For others, however, many years and perhaps even the rest of their lives will be spent in this phase, with their death ultimately being caused by something other than cancer.

Mullan and Hoffman (1990) divided the chronic stage of

cancer into two parts: (1) *extended survival*, when the person has completed treatments and resumes a more normal life but must deal with realistic fears of recurrence and (2) *permanent survival*, when people are considered to have been cured but still experience the physical and emotional impact of cancer, its changes, losses, barriers, and rewards. This chapter will focus on the chronic stage and will look at the impact cancer has on people in this phase and how psychotherapists can help them to make the most of the rest of their lives. The third phase of cancer, the *terminal stage* of the disease, involves the time when death from cancer seems inevitable. That phase has been discussed in the previous chapter.

Making the Transition to the Chronic Stage

The chronic stage of cancer is a time of uncertainty. Especially during the first few years after treatment, many people continue to feel a great deal of fear and apprehension. They may also be coping with long-term side effects of their treatments. Many cancer survivors who have had surgery, intensive chemotherapy, and radiotherapy report that it takes them a year to regain their energy, their ability to concentrate, and their sense of physical well-being. Most also gradually regain a sense of emotional well-being during that first year after treatment. According to Andersen (1992, p. 556), "Longitudinal data suggest that when localized disease is controlled and recovery proceeds unimpaired, the severe distress of diagnosis dissipates and emotions stabilize by one year posttreatment." Considerable improvement in mood is often evident as early as three or four months after treatment.

On the other hand, significant distress in response to the diagnosis of cancer may persist for years, particularly among people who had preexisting emotional disorders, surgery that altered physical appearance, or chemotherapy. One study found that 33 percent of women who had mastectomies still had severe mood disturbance two years after surgery (Edgar, Rosberger, & Nowlis,

1992) while 44 percent of women who had chemotherapy for breast cancer continued to experience disruption in their lives two years later (Haber, 1993). Research on how people cope with the chronic phase of cancer is limited and does not provide a good picture of that period (Hopwood & Maguire, 1992). Consequently, each person must be assessed individually and prolonged emotional distress should not be viewed as unusual or abnormal.

Passage Through the Chronic Stage

The general literature on how people cope with crises can shed some light on patterns that are probably typical of many people in the chronic stage of cancer. Spencer and Adams (1990), for example, described seven steps that characterize passage through a life crisis or transition. The first three—numbness, denial, and depression—usually occur during the initial or crisis stage of cancer. However, the next four steps may well reflect the experience of dealing with the chronic stage and are adapted below to describe cancer survivors in that stage:

Letting go of the past. People still feel fragile and may have considerable anxiety and depression but begin to have hope and to focus on the future. They often examine their past beliefs and assumptions and start to move toward a new normal. Support, sharing with peers, and relaxation are important during this stage as are self-care, exercise, and new activities to bolster energy and promote a forward momentum.

Testing the limits. The wish for reinvolvement strengthens, often with a sense of time urgency. Focus shifts from inner concerns to other people and activities. Assessing and building on strengths and interests, clarifying goals, and mentoring and peer support are useful during this stage.

Searching for meaning. During this stage, the sense of urgency diminishes and people achieve a greater sense of inner peace and direction. They can take pride in having dealt well with cancer. Some balance is attained as they rediscover the rewarding aspects of their lives before cancer and integrate them with new interests and activities. They may be more comfortable with themselves than ever before and place greater value on time alone and introspective activities such as journal writing and meditation.

Integration. People feel more grounded and optimistic about the future. Cancer recedes in importance in their lives and they feel ready to move on, often in new and more rewarding directions. One cancer survivor used the metaphor of a quilt to describe this process. When the diagnosis is first made, all squares in the quilt depict cancer. Over time, that changes until finally cancer becomes only one square in the quilt of a person's whole life. Confidence and a sense of control increase and relationships and interests are deepened. People even begin to see benefits from their experience with cancer.

Facilitating Movement Through the Steps

Movement through the steps in the chronic stage can be facilitated by helping cancer survivors look at the process they have been going through and assess how far they have come and where they want to be. Bouts with depression or anxiety can be normalized while focusing on successes in handling the crisis and redirecting energy. Reviewing past successes in negotiating transitions, exploring fears and ways to manage them, and setting goals can all increase energy and optimism. Techniques such as cognitive restructuring, assertiveness training, meditation, systematic desensitization, relaxation, and use of support systems are helpful in the chronic stage as they were in the crisis stage. Guilt and regrets may also need attention, as well as the negative impact of the disease on relationships.

Of course, not all cancer survivors move smoothly out of the crisis stage and into the chronic stage. Research shows that the emotional distress of people in the crisis phase of cancer is often concealed, overlooked, or neglected and that only a small percentage of people who would benefit from psychotherapy during that period actually receive help (Hopwood & Maguire, 1992). Although some people will regain emotional stability spontaneously over time, other will not.

People seen in psychotherapy during the chronic phase of cancer, then, probably will fall in one of three groups:

1.   People who began psychotherapy during the crisis phase of cancer and have continued in psychotherapy as they move into the chronic phase.

2.   People who have been highly distressed throughout the process of coping with cancer but who did not seek treatment until the chronic phase. They may have assumed their distress would diminish after treatment or may have focused so much on their physical needs that they neglected the emotional ones. They may have been referred to therapy by a physician or loved one who was concerned about their continued difficulty in managing their feelings, or the cancer survivor may be concerned about cancer-related issues such as sexual dysfunction or physical changes that may not have been attended to until the cancer treatments were over.

3.   People who have coped with cancer fairly well throughout the process but who are now questioning their goals and activities. They may seek therapy for help in understanding the changes their experience with cancer has precipitated in their values and outlook and in modifying their lives so they are more rewarding.

Common Issues for People in the Chronic Stage

Although all three groups of people have somewhat different needs and resources, several common issues are likely to arise for everyone in the chronic phase:

Making the transition from the crisis phase to the chronic phase. Most cancer survivors, of course, are relieved when treatments end and they resume a more normal life. However, fear often increases at that time because people have lost the security and protection afforded by their treatments and by frequent contact with their medical team. They may even fear thinking that they are cured lest this somehow magically cause a return of the disease once they have let their guard down.

Another common and difficult transition is the change from patient to well person. People may regret losing the special attention they had when they were undergoing treatment and may be surprised to find that others expect them to quickly resume their former activities and responsibilities while they are still reeling from the impact of cancer and its treatments. Brigham (1994, p. 60) described what she called the "Post-Recovery Existential Crisis," in which desired physical outcomes have occurred and people feel they should be happy but have a sense of emptiness and meaninglessness. This reaction is common at the conclusion of any challenging major endeavor such as writing a book or climbing a mountain but is particularly common in cancer survivors because, for most, they did not believe there would be a life after cancer. Now there is, and they are not sure what to do with it.

Cancer survivors, as well as their family and friends, may need help with these transitions. Most people will have been changed by their experience with cancer and, especially in the first few months after treatment, they will need time to make the transition, to cope with the physical and emotional aftermath of the disease, and to establish their identities as cancer survivors in the chronic phase. As Zimpfer (1992, p. 207) wrote, "Clients yearn to return to normal, but recognize eventually that only a new normal is possible." Psychotherapy can speed this transition and help reduce people's distress following cancer treatments.

Adaptation to changes in self-image. Part of the "new normal" experienced by many cancer survivors is a new sense of self. For most, this is a positive change, reflecting a sense of accomplishment and pride at having coped successfully with cancer. In the words of cancer survivors:

"I feel like I can do anything now. I'm a stronger person than I thought I was. Cancer is a growth experience."

"I'm proud that I faced a terrible illness with courage and determination. My experience with cancer raised my self-esteem because I feel that I conquered another obstacle in my life."

"I am proud that I kept my sense of humor and courage. Many people have told me what an inspiration I have been."

However, for some cancer survivors, the impact of cancer on self-esteem is negative: "I feel much more vulnerable. I feel like I don't know who I am any more. I trusted my body, I trusted myself, and then everything fell apart."

Although some cancer survivors may judge themselves harshly, themes of courage, strength, and determination arise even in those who feel distressed and depressed. Therapy can help people recognize and appreciate their success and enhance their self-esteem and self-efficacy.

Changes in goals and priorities. Priorities shift for many cancer survivors, with relationships, self-actualization, new experiences, and living life in a full and meaningful way typically becoming more important while details and possessions become less important. Again, the words of cancer survivors capture these changes well:

"It is no longer necessary for me to be perfect at work."

"I try to experience all I can and have new adventures whenever possible."

"The house doesn't have to be spotless all the time now."

"I had always wanted to play the organ. Well, now I am and I adore it."

"I don't worry so much about appearance. I am more concerned with people."

"I came from a poor family and my values were material. Now I value life, good health, a good night's sleep."

"Concerns I had prior to cancer have all been tempered, changed, or eradicated by dealing with cancer."

"I now do things that I enjoy like painting. I joined a community orchestra. I enjoy each day as it comes."

"Important to me now is living well and living peacefully, in harmony with me."

"My major goal no longer is to find a significant other. Now my major goal is to be significant."

"Before I had cancer, I didn't set goals. I just did whatever other people wanted me to do. Now I set goals. I learned to say no and to be selective."

Some people make dramatic changes in their lives after cancer. One woman left a successful and demanding career to stay home with her young child. One man left a job in business to begin training to become a counselor. Others become involved in volunteer work with cancer organizations, wanting to help people benefit from their experience with cancer and promote research on treatments for the disease. One woman who had breast cancer described her life now as absorbed with "pink ribbons and petitions."

Of course, not all people make such dramatic changes. Some develop a new appreciation for activities and relationships they had taken for granted and reinvest their energy with a freshness and excitement. Even children and adolescents who survive cancer show positive changes. Anholt, Fritz, and Keener (1993) compared cancer survivors between the ages of six and eighteen with their peers who had not had cancer. At an average of twenty months after completing treatment, the cancer survivors achieved significantly higher scores on intellectual self-concept, school status self-concept, behavior, and overall happiness, although their physical self-image was somewhat lower than those who had not had cancer. The young cancer survivors seemed to have a renewed appreciation for themselves and their lives and a greater sense of competence.

For nearly all cancer survivors, the disease serves as a turning point, a time to reassess their lives and either fulfill long-neglected goals or reinvest in an already rewarding life. "Cancer may have seemed to be the end for me—that was before. Cancer now seems to be more of a beginning—a place to launch from, learn from, improve from."

Changes in time perspective. Cancer increases people's awareness of their mortality and leads them to realize that their lives are finite. For some, this is discouraging: "I find myself identifying with my parents' generation—planning my death instead of thirty more years of life. I do not find any richness in this new perspective."

Even with an excellent prognosis, some continue to feel that death is imminent and avoid thoughts of the future: "I have lost my feeling that I will live forever. It's like losing your innocence."

"Any future plans have been shot. I'm afraid to make any plans, sometimes even for the next weekend."

"I feel real sorry for myself when I see others buying Christmas presents in July or talking about their vacations next year."

For others, the altered time perspective renews appreciation of the time left: "I accept my finality and am grateful for each day." Long-fantasized trips and once-enjoyed activities are pursued with a vengeance as people realize these goals cannot be deferred indefinitely. Involvement in new and challenging activities also seems to be a way for people to affirm that they are alive and healthy.

Changes in relationships. In the interpersonal area too, people seem to clarify their priorities, investing more in important relationships and discarding those that are unfulfilling. People who were not supportive or understanding during the crisis stage of cancer are often the first relationships to be eliminated. Cancer survivors also seem to become more accepting of the needs of others as well as more likely to express and value their own needs and importance in relationships.

"Now I'm more patient with my kids. I've come to accept each has his or her own destiny to live out."

"Two positive things that came out of my cancer were wonderful warm friendships with people in my support group like I never had before and the ability to cry and confide my worries and fears to others."

"I used to value a normal sex life. I miss it, but now I value other parts of our relationship much more."

"I work harder at keeping the important ties stronger and alive. I've given up negative people in my life with no regrets."

"Cancer made us realize you can't take things for granted. My family never hangs up the phone now without saying, 'I love you.'"

Roles change along with relationships. Here too, people place more emphasis on their inner needs and values, on doing what is important to them rather than acting to please others: "I never thought of myself before. I was always somebody's wife or mother or daughter, but now I can integrate: I can be some of those things but also just be myself."

Changes in assumptions about oneself and the world. For most cancer survivors, life has become less predictable and more finite. Self-reliance is more important, and good relationships often become more central. Religious and spiritual beliefs may change in either direction. One cancer survivor wrote, "I expected my faith to kick in magically but it didn't. I haven't been to church since my diagnosis," while another said, "I listen to the voice of God in the sights, sounds, and smells of nature. It helps me to place myself and my condition in perspective." People seem to feel freer to be themselves and have discarded many of their earlier fears: "I used to be afraid of the dark, of death, of being alone. Now I don't have a fear of anything. I am free for the first time in my life." However, new fears, especially the fear of recurrence, may be strong.

Establishing a healthier lifestyle. Many cancer survivors are eager to improve their physical and emotional health. They seek to regain the vigor they felt before their treatments, to reduce the impact of physical changes that have resulted from their treatments, and perhaps to ward off a recurrence of cancer. Appropriate weight loss, increased exercise, dietary changes, and use of vitamins are common approaches to improved health. In addition, some cancer survivors continue psychotherapy, meditation, relaxation, and other coping skills they learned in the process of dealing with cancer.

Nearly all cancer survivors I have worked with view themselves as having gone through a journey, filled with pain and upset but also with discovery and growth. They are eager to tell their story, and this seems to be healing. Support groups, journal writing, and renewal of close relationships have a particularly important role for the person who is making the transition from the crisis to the extended survival phase. Therapy too can be a place for people to review their journey, to make sense of it, and to integrate it with their other life experiences so that it ceases to be all-consuming.

Promoting a Positive Emotional Stance

Promoting a positive emotional stance in cancer survivors in the chronic stage is important for several reasons. Hardiness, characterized by control, commitment, and challenge, has been associated with better health outcomes and can decrease one's chance of becoming ill by as much as 50 percent (Kobasa, 1979; Witmer & Sweeney, 1992; see Chapter One for further discussion). Although little research has focused directly on the relationship between hardiness and the aftermath of cancer, it is reasonable to believe that an attitude of hardiness is associated with continuing to be free of signs of cancer as well as with successfully regaining energy and physical well-being. An attitude of hardiness can help people deal more successfully with the negative impact cancer may have had on their functioning, appearance, and relationships. It also can help people cope with stress and maintain good immune system functioning.

Siebert (1993) described the survivor personality as having the following ten characteristics:

1. Empathy for others, including those with whom we disagree

2. Ability to see patterns in relationships

3. Ability to make good use of one's own intuition

4. Ability to anticipate the future and take appropriate action

5. A sense of individualism

6. Feeling comfortable in complex or threatening situations

7. Optimism and self-confidence

8. Viewing new unanticipated or unpleasant experiences as challenges

9. Being able to transform problems or misfortunes into something positive

10. Improved sense of well-being and enjoyment with age

These ten characteristics incorporate the features of the hardy personality and present a model for healthy functioning in the chronic stage of dealing with cancer. This model can be discussed with clients and ways developed to help them achieve the qualities delineated in Siebert's model.

Cancer as an Opportunity to Review and Improve One's Life

At least half of those people who are successfully treated for cancer report some positive benefit from their disease (Barraclough, 1994). One study of women who had breast cancer provided a "unanimous report of the positive impact of the breast cancer experience. . . . They reported a revaluing of their lives and a reprioritization of their expenditure of personal time and energy . . ." (Westlake & Selder, 1990, p. 130). Rolland (1994) observed that cancer survivors' brush with death helps them to clarify what is meaningful and important to them. As one survivor put it, "Cancer has been a huge wake-up call." Siegel (1993, p. xvii) too emphasized the power of cancer to improve one's life and serve as a new beginning: "For some of you, learning that you are mortal finally gives you permission to live your life."

Triumphing over cancer can enhance self-esteem, provide a clear sense of priorities, and promote awareness and appreciation of life. People often develop a better capacity to live in the present and become more inner directed. They typically are eager to make sense of their past experiences and move on to a better future. Many cancer survivors experience fundamental changes, sometimes small but sometimes dramatic, as a result of cancer. Zimpfer (1992, p. 207) described these changes as follows: "Transformations may come slowly and painfully, or can be almost instantaneous; in any case they are the real stuff of renewal of life, potentiating healing forces and switching off destructive ones."

Siegel (1993) placed considerable emphasis on the symbolic meaning of cancer in a person's life. He suggested asking what cancer gave a person permission to do and using that information as a cue to feelings and wants. I have not always found this line of inquiry to be productive, and unless pursued carefully it can raise guilt and blame. However, it may be a useful perspective to help some people reevaluate the direction of their lives.

Cancer survivors' foreshortened time perspective can also be used in a positive way to help people determine what is important for them to accomplish or experience in the next six months or a year. Identification and realization of dreams and hopes can help people move beyond cancer to a new appreciation of life. In this and in many other ways, psychotherapy can help cancer survivors find even more happiness and rewards from their lives after cancer than they did before cancer.

Dealing with the Long-Term Impact of Cancer

In order to change their lives for the better, people need to deal with the residues of their disease, the physical, psychological, spiritual, social, and financial changes (Doka, 1993). Some goals may change out of necessity rather than choice—for example, if cancer has impaired ability to bear children or return to a former job. Those changes must be addressed. Decisions still may need to be made about cosmetic or reconstructive surgery and about the use of prostheses. These decisions too need to be integrated into the person's overall goals and self-image. Unfinished business may remain with the medical team and with family and friends; disappointments, appreciations, and questions need to be identified and expressed in constructive ways.

Despite their foreshortened time perspective, cancer survivors need to take time to heal and move on rather than rush into rapid and extreme changes. They need to determine what to leave behind, what they can learn from their disease, and what they want to add to their lives.

Psychotherapy can help people to review their decisions and ensure that they are thoughtful and realistic. Plans can be developed to take small, safe, manageable steps that will reduce inertia and create a sense of movement. Ceremonies and rituals can be useful in marking important transitions such as the end of chemotherapy, having enough hair to discard one's wigs, and anniversaries since diagnosis. Agnetti and Young (1993) suggested the use of metaphors of newness, birth, and change as well as time-contrasting questions such as "How are you feeling now compared with how you felt in the middle of your treatments?" as ways of promoting optimism and a sense of progress.

Coping with Fear, Uncertainty, and Self-Blame

One of the unfortunate legacies of cancer is a continuing fear of recurrence that affects nearly all cancer survivors. Macaskill and Monach (1990) called this the Damocles Syndrome, plaguing not only the survivors but their families and loved ones as well. They have been shaken by one bout with cancer and feel vulnerable and uncertain about the future. Their bodies have already let them down once and therefore they may no longer trust them.

Especially in the first year after treatment, recurrence feels almost inevitable, even for people with a positive prognosis. Women who had breast cancer, for example, spend at least five years being hypervigilant and fearful about the return of cancer (Haber, 1993).

Fears of recurrence have many triggers:

• The end of treatments or of frequent visits to physicians may leave some feeling vulnerable and unprotected.

• Minor physical symptoms such as a cough, a headache or other unexplained pain, changes in bowel habits, or fatigue lead cancer survivors to worry that the disease has returned or metastasized.

• Medical checkups, frequent during the first year or two after cancer, raise fears.

• Anniversaries, such as the date cancer was initially diagnosed, a birthday, the anniversary of a parent's death, or the time when the survivor reaches the age when a relative died of cancer, are reminders of mortality and of the disease.

• Deaths of others from cancer, either acquaintances or famous people, increase fear and apprehension. Clients of mine who admired Jacqueline Kennedy were upset by her death; they seemed to believe that if even she could not marshal the resources to fight cancer successfully, there was little hope that they could survive the disease.

• Many cancer survivors have idiosyncratic reminders of their disease. One woman received her diagnosis shortly before a scheduled vacation to the beach that was canceled so that she could have surgery. Thereafter, trips to the beach were filled with apprehension and worry.

Cancer survivors are beset by both anticipated and unanticipated fears. As one cancer survivor said, "My fears are triggered by reading an article, hearing something, passing the hospital where I had my surgery. At other times, they just come out of the blue." Sometimes these fears are so great that they cause people to avoid medical checkups, ignore symptoms, and withdraw from rewarding activities that are associated with cancer. Even peer support groups may be shunned because members who are dealing with recurrences serve as reminders of what might happen.

Although fear is probably the most troubling feeling to result from cancer, other issues also may arise. Some people blame themselves for their disease and in fact a clear connection sometimes does seem to be present between cancer and behaviors. People who smoke cigarettes and subsequently develop lung cancer are an example. Although therapists may need to agree that people's previous behaviors were not ideal, emphasis should be on what can be done differently now rather than on what was done wrong.

People may find that others avoid them and treat them differently. One woman in a visible and powerful position was put behind the scenes because her supervisor thought that her gaunt appearance and hair loss detracted from her credibility. A man was denied a renewal of a long-term consulting contract because his employer feared he might not live long enough to fulfill the terms of the contract.

Family relationships often shift in the aftermath of cancer. Sometimes a partner's difficulty in dealing with cancer may lead to the end of a marriage. One woman who previously had been reluctant to confront her husband's drug use had no difficulty expressing herself when she learned he had used up medication that had been prescribed to relieve her pain. Siblings as well as spouses may still be suffering from the loss of attention that resulted when a child was diagnosed with cancer. Parents who have had cancer and are fearful that they may not live to see their children grow up may pressure their children to achieve milestones that are premature or beyond their abilities. People need help in coping with these feelings and experiences effectively.

In addition to techniques discussed elsewhere in this book, the following approaches can be helpful:

- Provide opportunity for expression of feelings.
- Normalize feelings, especially fears of recurrence, self-blame, longing for the past, anger, and a sense of urgency.

- At the same time, help people find positive and constructive ways to address those feelings, using both cognitive restructuring and behavioral change.
- Help people recognize the impact cancer has had on their relationships and enable them to make thoughtful and gradual changes, using assertion and sound communication skills rather than angry and impulsive relationship changes.
- Provide support and empathy.
- Promote skills and behaviors that will lead to the development of healthier attitudes and habits.
- Facilitate the use of role models, peer support, and success stories; these can be both empowering and encouraging during this stage.
- Psychodynamic psychotherapy, usually minimized during the crisis stage of cancer, now may help people cope with old losses and concerns that resurfaced during the diagnosis and treatment of cancer; it may also help change long-term self-defeating patterns. This process can contribute to the development of a sense of growth and progress after cancer and can help people reduce the importance cancer has in their lives.
- Help people develop strategies for dealing with their fears of recurrence. Such strategies may include affirmations, distraction, and the decision to consult a physician for all physical symptoms that last more than one week. Having plans to cope with fears can be reassuring and brings the fears under control.
- Help people identify the strengths they demonstrated in their fight against cancer so that they can take pride in those strengths.

Establishing a Healthier Lifestyle

In 1979, the United States Public Health Service reported that at least 53 percent of the deaths in the United States were caused by "life-style and self-destructive and negligent behavior" (Witmer & Sweeney, 1992, p. 140). A final step in working with people in the survival stages of cancer is helping them develop a healthier lifestyle. This can promote a sense of emotional well-being and self-esteem, reduce the likelihood of another episode of cancer as well as of other illnesses, and enable people to cope effectively with future crises. It also can reduce their tendency to blame themselves for their disease and promote feelings of control, self-efficacy, and empowerment.

Careful planning of lifestyle changes is important to promote motivation and involvement. Without adequate support and planning, involvement in healthy activities may not be maintained. Lewis, Sperry, and Carlson (1993), for example, reported that 50 percent of people who embark on exercise programs drop out of those programs within six months. Zimpfer (1992) recommended that cancer survivors establish a two-year health plan in which people initiate changes one at a time, adding a new focus every few months, while reevaluating and modifying old behaviors. This approach not only promotes a healthier lifestyle but gives an optimistic message about health and survival. Barriers to involvement in lifestyle changes should be anticipated and addressed while expectations of accomplishment and success are encouraged. Extreme or unrealistic goals should be modified; people are more likely to be motivated by achieving goals that are within their reach than by failing to reach goals that are too high. Slips and deviations from plans are to be expected, and people should be accepting of their own inconsistency.

Encouraging people to follow the guidelines below is likely to help them establish a healthier lifestyle in the aftermath of cancer:

1.   Clarify and act according to one's spiritual and philosophical beliefs, whether they include formal religion, good works, love of nature, commitment to family, or other important values.

2.   Maintain balance in one's life, so that work and play, challenge and fun, the intellectual and the physical combine in a rewarding whole.

3. Learn from the past and plan for and look forward to the future, but live in the present with mindfulness and appreciation.

4. Minimize stress, fatigue, and anxiety and use effective coping mechanisms to deal with them when they occur; obtain seven to eight hours of restful sleep nightly.

5. Maintain positive self-esteem, a sense of control over one's life, and an internal locus of control.

6. Build on positive emotions such as joy, peace, and enthusiasm; express and modify emotions such as depression, anxiety, and anger. Laughter and a sense of humor are likely to promote relaxation and a sense of well-being.

7. Engage in regular exercise, ideally at least three times a week for twenty minutes (Lewis, Sperry, & Carlson, 1993).

8. Follow a healthy diet that will lead to maintenance of an appropriate weight. Eat regular, healthy meals that are low in fat, sugar, caffeine, and sodium and high in grains, fruits, and vegetables. Cruciferous vegetables such as cabbage, broccoli, brussels sprouts, and cauliflower, in particular, have been associated with low rates of cancer (Winograd, 1992). Consume ample quantities of water or other healthy liquids daily. As recommended by physicians, use nutritional supplements such as beta-carotene or selenium, which are associated with a reduced incidence of cancer.

9. Abstain from smoking and make minimal use of alcohol.

10. Have a rewarding, challenging, and interesting focus to life, whether it is work, child rearing, homemaking, education, volunteer work, or leisure activities. According to Witmer and Sweeney (1992), job satisfaction is related to hardiness, and one of the best predictors of longevity is satisfaction with one's work.

11. Maintain close, loving relationships that provide support, sharing, and a sense of belonging. Witmer and Sweeney (1992, p. 145) reported that "trust, intimacy, caring, companionship, compassion, and similar qualities of a loving relationship promote good health and longevity."

12. Establish a routine that promotes relaxation and self-

expression. This may include meditation, mental imagery, writing, or other activities that are personally rewarding.

Overview of Chapter

Clearly, psychotherapists can contribute a great deal to people in the survival or chronic stages of cancer. What initially seemed like a devastating and terrifying experience can be transformed into one that leads to growth, health, and joy. In the words of a cancer survivor, "I am proud that I did not ever give up, that I faced cancer, that cancer could not stop me, my spirit, my love of life, and that cancer could be for me a place to learn, an impetus for improvement and growth."

Resource A: Six-Session Counseling Framework

. . . .

The following is a tentative outline for individual counseling with an adult cancer survivor seen shortly after the diagnosis has been made. Each session may be spread out over several meetings, depending on the needs of the client. Worksheets, included in the next section, can be incorporated into the treatment to provide focus and tasks to be completed between sessions as well as a sense of accomplishment.

Before the first session begins, a brief written questionnaire is given to the person to obtain demographic data: name and address, birth date, person to contact in case of an emergency, occupation, medical diagnosis and date determined, brief history of medical and psychological treatment, names and ages of immediate family members or close friends, and names of physicians.

Session 1: Understanding the Person with Cancer

The purpose of the first session is to understand the person and the diagnosis and to put them in context. Particular attention should be paid to identifying coping skills and support systems. Although most of the session will be devoted to information gathering and exploration of feelings and reactions, the person should be left with some tool or plan at the end of the session to initiate progress and instill feelings of hope. The following is a tentative outline and suggested dialogue for the first session.

I. Understanding the diagnosis and the person's reactions to the diagnosis

A. I understand you've recently been diagnosed with cancer. Tell me about that. (People usually will tell their story, including the initial symptoms, medical visits and tests, anxiety prior to the diagnosis, how the final diagnosis was determined and delivered, and reactions to that information. Any of these pieces that are omitted can be elicited through questioning.)

B. What has it been like for you to know that you have cancer?

C. What feelings and concerns has it brought up for you?

D. What have you done to help yourself handle this information?

E. What family and friends are aware that you have been diagnosed with cancer? How have they reacted?

F. What information have your physicians given you about your disease? Your treatment options? The prognosis for your disease?

G. What decisions have you had to consider?

H. What does all this mean to you?

II. Putting the reactions in context

A. It would help me to understand the present situation if I had some information about your life before the diagnosis. (This transition helps people feel comfortable about shifting their focus away from the disease.)

B. Tell me what your life was like before you learned you had cancer. (Questioning should elicit information about the nature and quality of support systems, occupational and leisure activities, concurrent stressors, spiritual activities and beliefs, mood and personality, cognitive abilities, prior health, resources and responsibilities.)

C. I'm sure we'll talk more about this later, but now I'd like to learn something about your background. (Questioning can touch on such areas as ethnic, sociocultural, and family background; education; relationships; and employment history. The goals of this area of inquiry include greater understanding of the person, particularly strengths and potential difficulties, and identification of areas that warrant further exploration because of their relevance to the person's reactions to the diagnosis of cancer.)

III. Assessing past coping skills

A. Have you or anyone you have been close to dealt with cancer before this? Tell me about that.
B. What other serious medical problems have you or people close to you dealt with?
C. At what other times in your life have you had to deal with very challenging or difficult situations? How did you react to those situations? How did you try to improve or resolve those situations? What approaches seemed to work best for you?

IV. Understanding the meaning cancer has for the person

A. I appreciate your filling me in on your background. It will help me to determine the best way for us to help you cope with your disease and its treatment. (This links the past to the presenting problem and makes clear that although the focus of treatment will be on coping with cancer, information on other aspects of the person's life can facilitate the therapy. This intervention also communicates a spirit of optimism and collaboration.)
B. How do you explain why you have cancer? (This explores the meaning the person has made of the disease.)

C. What are the next steps you have to take in addressing your disease and its treatment? What concerns do you have about those steps? (This elicits information about decisions that must be made or treatment that is anticipated.)

D. So far, what has been the hardest part of having been diagnosed with cancer? What do you think might make recovery difficult? (These questions, as well as the previous one, can facilitate goal setting.)

V. Promoting involvement, hope, and self-efficacy

A. Therapists have found that helping people with cancer explore and maybe make some changes in their feelings, their thoughts, and their behaviors really can make a difference in how they cope with the disease. Therapy can help you reduce depression and anxiety related to the disease; make decisions about treatment; handle some of the side effects of treatment; communicate better with family, friends, and physicians; and maybe even improve the functioning of your immune system. (Emphasize those potential goals that seem most likely to be important to the person.) Worksheet 4 might be useful at this point.

B. (Therapist now would provide a brief description of cognitive-behavioral and other interventions that have been shown to be effective in helping people cope with cancer.)

C. What other information would you like about my work with people with cancer?

D. How do you feel about our working together to help you cope with your disease and its treatment?

E. If person is willing to become involved in psychotherapy, session can be concluded with the following steps:

1. If indicated, administer checklists such as the Beck

Depression Inventory or the Profile of Mood States discussed in Chapter Three of this book to provide further information on the person's emotional state.

2. Teach and practice a simple approach to relaxation such as deep breathing; this will begin to give the person some control over anxiety.

3. Suggest a relatively brief, easy task for the person to do such as reading the first chapter of a recommended book, beginning a diary of experiences with cancer and its treatments, listing times between now and the next appointment when the person feels particularly distressed, telling a friend about the diagnosis, completing Worksheet 1 in Resource B, or making a list of questions the person has about the disease. Such tasks can promote involvement in therapy, increase feelings of control and self-efficacy, and provide a jumping-off point for the next therapy session.

4. Obtain a clear picture of the person's medical appointments and treatment between this session and the next one. If necessary, help person develop questions for those appointments and process any immediate decisions that must be made. If appropriate, offer a supportive telephone call (for example, after surgery, after the first chemotherapy treatment).

5. Schedule the next appointment.

Session 2: Introduction of Cognitive and Behavioral Strategies

The purpose of this session is to initiate development of coping skills that will reduce depression, facilitate decision making, and help the person deal effectively with the stress of cancer and its treatments.

I.   Session generally should begin by providing some opportunity for the person to express feelings, to discuss tasks that were completed between sessions, and to process the events of the week that are relevant to coping with cancer.

II. The primary focus of this session is initiating the teaching of cognitive-behavioral techniques that will promote coping. The specific techniques that are presented depend on the needs of the client and the preferences of the therapist. For people who recently have been diagnosed, important interventions usually include the following:

   A. Systematic decision making
   B. Identification of troubling cognitive distortions related to cancer and ways to dispute them
   C. Relaxation, usually progressive muscle relaxation
   D. Meditation and visualization
   E. Development of support systems, either by joining a peer support group for people with cancer or by drawing on natural support systems

III. Tasks between sessions generally should be suggested to implement the skills that have been taught. If the person feels ready, he or she might be encouraged to list upsetting feelings that arise, the circumstances of those feelings, and the cognitions behind the feelings. The person also might begin to dispute those cognitions. Worksheet 2 might be used at this point.

Session 3: Facilitating the Use of Support Systems

Sessions 2 and 3 may be reversed, combined, or scheduled close together, depending on the needs and availability of the client and the people in the client's support system. Session 3 entails meeting with the client and any friends or family members that the person identifies as providing essential support and/or needing some help themselves. This would usually include the spouse or significant

other. Meetings with children, parents, or siblings may also be helpful at this time or may be scheduled for a later date. Goals of this
session include promoting open and honest communication
between cancer survivor and support system, helping people in the
support system deal with their own anxiety and upset, and determining ways for the people in the support system to help the
cancer survivor without overtaxing themselves. Worksheet 3 can
be used as part of this session.

Session 4: Solidifying Coping Skills

This session is designed to solidify coping skills that have been presented in earlier sessions, such as disputing cognitive distortions,
and to add new skills to the person's repertoire. Medical treatments
probably have begun by this time and should be addressed in psychotherapy. Steps in this session might include the following:

I.   Processing feelings, decisions, and important events since the
     previous session

II. Following up on tasks suggested for completion between ses-
     sions

III. Continuing to pay attention to disputing cognitive distortions
     and replacing them with cognitions that are more likely to
     promote optimism and a fighting spirit

IV. Building on relaxation skills that already have been taught by
     adding guided imagery to the client's repertoire of skills, possi-
     bly focusing on coping with surgery, building up the immune
     system, reducing the side effects of chemotherapy, or other
     needs or concerns of the client

V.   Continuing to promote good use of support systems

VI. Again, establishing tasks between sessions that build on skills
     (at this point, a plan to meditate on a regular basis often is
     indicated and can be implemented between sessions)

Session 5: Dealing with Medical Treatments

The exact nature of this session depends on what medical treatments are underway, how they are affecting the person, and how successful the person has been at disputing cognitive distortions and implementing a program of relaxation and meditation. The overall goal of this session is to ensure the implementation of coping skills that have been taught in earlier sessions and to promote their effective use.

This session also may be a time to begin to direct people's attention to other aspects of their lives. If surgery has been completed and people are in the process of receiving chemotherapy or radiotherapy, they probably will benefit not only from help in dealing with those treatments and their impact but also in resuming some of the rewarding parts of their lives. Continued involvement with supportive friends and family is one way to increase activities. In addition, this session might revisit the person's life before cancer in order to identify activities that are likely to be realistic and rewarding. Particularly beneficial are activities that promote feelings of pleasure as well as mastery or competence.

Session 6: Reinforcing and Building on Gains

If the person has responded well to psychotherapy and is making good use of the coping skills that have been developed through therapy, if support systems are in place and are offering needed help and caring, and if the client's medical treatments are going smoothly, the client might be ready to complete therapy with this session. Others, who continue to be depressed over their diagnosis and its treatment and who are not yet making good use of cognitive and behavioral techniques, may need to continue weekly psychotherapy until those goals have been achieved. A third group, comprised of people who have coped fairly well with cancer and its treatments but who still need some help with their own motivation and their moods, may be seen on a less frequent basis, perhaps every two weeks or once a month until they have completed their medical treatments and returned as fully as possible to their work, home, and leisure activities. Yet another group of people may be coping well with cancer but may want to continue therapy in order to take a look at their lives and their goals in an effort to establish a more rewarding and meaningful lifestyle. Whether psychotherapy is continued beyond this session and what the schedule of psychotherapy should be will be determined by the needs of the clients, their progress thus far, their medical treatments and physical condition, and their interest in continued help.

As psychotherapy approaches its final phase, whether that occurs at the sixth session or later, the following goals will usually be on the agenda:

- Review of the person's psychotherapy
- Further attention to the person's interpretation of cancer and its existential impact, ensuring that the person has accepted and integrated the diagnosis and is dealing successfully with any spiritual, value-related, or other issues that have been raised by the diagnosis
- Encouragement of continued involvement with support systems, with attention paid to any interpersonal conflicts as well as any help that might be needed with communication and assertiveness skills
- Continued use of cognitive restructuring to promote optimism and reduce depression
- Continued use of relaxation, meditation, visualization, and other techniques that have been developed to reduce anxiety and the side effects of treatment as well as bolster the immune system
- Exploration of the impact of the temporary and permanent physical changes that have been caused by cancer and its treatment and use of interventions to help people cope with those changes
- Establishment of a healthy and rewarding lifestyle, with plans being made to incorporate exercise, nutritional eating, stress management, and other beneficial activities into the person's life

- Alerting people to the common difficulties that may develop after the cancer treatments have been completed, such as fear of recurrence, the need for a new normal, and changes in relationships and values, as well as giving them some guidelines for coping with those concerns
- Reinforcement of the person's accomplishments and strengths, as well as development of a plan to continue to use effective coping skills and build on those strengths
- Planning for follow-up, either in person or via telephone, and assurance that the psychotherapist can be consulted again in the future if difficulties arise that seem amenable to psychotherapy

Worksheets 5 and 6 facilitate accomplishment of the goals in this session.

Resource B: Worksheets to Facilitate Psychotherapy

Worksheet 1: Writing About My Diagnosis

1. What are your most vivid memories about learning that you had cancer?
2. What were your thoughts and feelings when you first learned of your diagnosis?
3. How have those thoughts and feelings changed?
4. What has helped you to cope with the diagnosis and manage your feelings?
5. How can others help you cope with your diagnosis?

Worksheet 2: Ways to Help Myself Cope with Cancer

The following is a list of many of the ways people have helped themselves cope with cancer. Review this list and select at least two of these activities that you think might help you at the present time. We will be discussing many of the approaches in this list during your therapy in order to help you deal successfully with cancer and its treatments.

Supportive Relationships

1. Join a support group, provide and accept support.
2. Make use of your natural support systems.
3. Use your experience and knowledge to help others.
4. Discuss your thoughts and feelings about cancer with someone you trust.
5. Spend time with a friend or a potential friend.
6. Ask someone for help.
7. Improve your relationship and communication with your spouse or partner.

Medical Help

1. Consult with a physician on a medical problem or question.
2. Get a medical evaluation or test.
3. Obtain the medical treatments you need, even though they may be difficult.
4. Make a list of questions you have for your physician.
5. Express yourself more directly to your physician.
6. Read a book or do some research on a medical question that concerns you.

Physical Health

1. Begin or continue an exercise program.

2. Improve your eating habits.

3. Take steps to maintain or achieve a healthy weight.

4. Stop smoking.

5. Reduce or eliminate alcohol consumption.

6. Improve your sleeping habits.

Relaxation and Imagery

1. Develop or continue a program of meditation.

2. Begin, maintain, or increase involvement in a rewarding leisure activity.

3. Make regular use of systematic relaxation.

4. Make regular use of visualization.

5. Increase your involvement in prayer, religion, or spirituality.

6. Take a relaxing and rewarding trip or vacation.

7. Become more involved in an expressive art.

8. Get a massage.

Emotional Health

1. Begin or continue psychotherapy.

2. Develop your assertiveness skills.

3. Develop your communication skills.

4. Begin or continue work on past issues that have been troubling you.

5. Maintain a journal or write about your thoughts, feelings, and experiences related to cancer.

6. Use cognitive restructuring to help yourself reduce anxiety and guilt.

7. Do something you have always wanted to do but never did.

8. Try to make each day a good one.

9. Deal more directly with your fears and problems.

10. Bring some humor and fun into your life.

11. Use positive affirmations on a regular basis.

12. Focus on your strengths rather than your shortcomings.

Your Own Approaches to Helping Yourself Cope with Cancer

1.

2.

3.

Worksheet 3: Facilitating Difficult Conversations About Cancer

General guidelines:

1. Use "I" statements.

2. Show empathy or understanding toward others.

3. Ask open questions, such as "How do you feel about this?" If that does not work, try multiple choice questions—for example, "Does this make you feel scared or angry or maybe just sad?"

4. Don't push—if talking feels bogged down, tense, or uncomfortable, table the conversation: "This is hard to talk about. Why don't we have dinner and maybe we can get back to this later?"

5. Do be assertive.

Talking with children (and others who may need gentle handling):

1. Tell the truth, simply and clearly.

2. Provide realistic reassurance—for example, "Mommy has very good doctors and they know the best medicines to use for cancer. I'm going to take all my medication and do everything I can to get well."

3. Ask for their feelings and thoughts.

4. If none are offered, guess at their feelings to give them permission to express negative thoughts—for example, "It must be pretty scary for you to hear that I'm sick."

5. If there still is no response, follow up later with an invitation to talk further: "I wonder if you have had a chance to think about what I told you this morning? What reactions have you had to my having cancer?"

6. Offer help with feelings, such as, "What would help you feel less scared?"

7. Look for indirect expressions of emotions: changes in usual mood, hostility toward others, acting out, relevant dreams and fantasies, changes in eating or sleeping, and so on. Make these topics for discussion.

8. Involve children and significant others in major decisions and transition points. Keep them informed and give them some choices and sense of control—for example, "Would you like to come with me when I get my treatment or would you rather go to the cafeteria with Mom?"

Talking with people who deny the seriousness of your disease:

1. Be sure that you have a realistic picture of your condition.

2. Plan and rehearse a three-part statement: Empathy, "I" statement, Request. Example: "I know it's hard for you to think about my having cancer, but it's very hard on me to keep my feelings bottled up and to make believe nothing is wrong. It would mean a lot to me if we could talk more openly about my condition."

3. Listen to the response, show understanding.

4. Stress the importance of your relationship with the person and try to find a mutually agreeable compromise such as "I don't want to talk about cancer all the time either and I do want to be optimistic, but when I really get scared, I need to talk to someone and you're the person I feel closest to."

5. Schedule a follow-up conversation: "Maybe we can talk more about this next week when you take me to the doctor."

6. Don't give up. At the same time, find other people you can talk with easily.

Worksheet 4: Qualities and Life Circumstances That May Be Associated with Prognosis

Associated with a negative prognosis:

1. Type C personality: Characterized by suppression and over-control of emotions, especially anger, passivity, compliance, and conformity.

2. Depressive symptoms: Feelings of hopelessness and helplessness. A negative mood may suppress antibodies that fight disease.

3. Acute, uncontrollable stress: This increases production of adrenaline and cortisol, which inhibit the immune system. Controllable stress does not have the same negative impact.

Associated with a positive prognosis:

1. Fighting spirit and a sense of optimism

2. Hardiness:

   Commitment or involvement in life

   Sense of control over one's life

   Sense of challenge, a belief that life's changes stimulate personal growth

3. Perceived social support, involving trust, intimacy, caring, companionship, understanding, and compassion, found to increase natural killer cell activity in people with cancer

   What can you do to develop qualities in yourself that are associated with a positive prognosis and reduce those that are associated with a negative prognosis?

Worksheet 5: Coping with the Fear of Recurrence or Treatment Failure

1. Fears come in waves; figure out the cause of each wave of fear. Possibilities:

   Anniversary of diagnosis, death of loved one, or other important event

   Illness of friend or family member

   Disturbing information

   Life change, such as divorce, vacation, promotion

   Change in treatment

   Physical symptoms

   Impending medical visit or test

   Death of another

2. Ways to address fears; choose approaches that address the cause of your fears:

   Affirmations

   Program of stress management, meditation, or relaxation

   Information gathering

   Talking with a friend or family member

   Taking a positive step (for example, celebrating the anniversary of your diagnosis, reaching out to a sick person)

   Distracting activity that absorbs you and focuses your attention

   Getting medical reassurance

   Internal conversation that addresses your cognitive distortions

   Visualization, talking with inner guide

   Avoiding source of the fear, if to do so is not self-destructive

3. Ways to address fears sparked by physical symptoms:

   Decide how long to wait before getting medical advice.

   Remind yourself of other possible explanations.

   Focus on the positive.

   Use coping mechanisms from the above section.

   If the symptom is not gone by the deadline you have set, obtain full and reliable medical information and tests.

Worksheet 6: Goal Setting

1. List three to five accomplishments that have been important to you.

2. What personal strengths and abilities helped you to overcome obstacles and accomplish these goals?

3. List two goals you have but have not yet achieved.

4. What has prevented you from achieving these goals?

5. What are the first steps you can take toward achieving these goals?

6. When will you take those steps?

7. Develop a detailed plan for the next year that will help you to maintain a healthy and rewarding lifestyle.

Resource C: Recommended Readings

An asterisk indicates resources that are especially useful.

For Therapists

Advances: The Journal of Mind-Body Health: all issues, but especially summer 1994, vol. 10, no. 3.

*Barraclough, J. (1994). *Cancer and emotion*. New York: Wiley.

Bernstein, J., & Rudman, M. (1989). *Books to help children cope with separation and loss: An annotated bibliography*. New Providence, N.J.: Bowker.

*Blitzer, A., Kutscher, A. H., Klagsbrun, S. C., De Bellis, R., Selder, F. E., Seeland, I. B., & Siegel, M. (Eds.). (1990). *Communicating with cancer patients and their families*. Philadelphia: Charles Press.

*Breitbart, W., & Holland, J. C. (Eds.). (1993). *Psychiatric aspects of symptom management in cancer patients*. Washington, D.C.: American Psychiatric Press.

CA: A Cancer Journal for Clinicians: all issues.

*Cooper, C. L., & Watson, M. (Eds.). (1991). *Cancer and stress: Psychological, biological and coping studies*. New York: Wiley.

Fawzy, F. I., & Morton, D. (1990). A structured psychiatric intervention for cancer patients. *Archives of General Psychiatry, 47*(8), 729–735.

*Golden, W. L., Gersh, W. D., & Robbins, D. M. (1992). *Psychological treatment of cancer patients*. Needham Heights, Mass.: Allyn & Bacon.

*Haber, S. (Ed.). (1993). *Breast cancer: A psychological treatment manual*. Phoenix: Division of Independent Practice.

Journal of Psychosocial Oncology: all issues.

McDaniel, S. H., Hepworth, J., & Doherty, W. (1992). *Medical family therapy*. New York: Basic Books.

Meichenbaum, D. (1985). *Stress inoculation training*. Elmsford, N.Y.: Pergamon Press.

*Moorey, S., & Greer, S. (1989). *Psychological therapy for patients with cancer: A new approach*. Washington, D.C.: American Psychiatric Press.

Rando, T. (Ed.). (1986). *Parental loss of a child*. Champaign, Ill.: Research Press.

*Rolland, J. S. (1994). *Families, illness, and disability*. New York: Basic Books.

Rosen, E. J. (1990). *Families facing death*. Lexington, Mass.: Lexington Books.

Rossi, E. L. (1993). *The psychobiology of mind-body healing*. New York: Norton.

Schlossberg, N. K. (1984). *Counseling adults in transition*. New York: Springer.

Spiegel, D. (1992). Effects of psychosocial support on patients with metastatic breast cancer. *Journal of Psychosocial Oncology, 10*(2), 113–120.

*Temoshok, L., & Dreher, H. (1992). *The Type C connection.* New York: Random House.

Walsh, F., & McGoldrick, M. (1991). *Living beyond loss.* New York: Norton.

Zimpfer, D. G. (1992). Psychosocial treatment of life-threatening disease: A wellness model. *Journal of Counseling and Development, 71*(2), 203–209.

For Therapists and Cancer Survivors

*Borysenko, J. (1988). *Minding the body, mending the mind.* New York: Bantam Books.

*Brigham, D. D. (1994). *Imagery for getting well.* New York: Norton.

Coping: a magazine about living with cancer that can be ordered through *Coping,* 2019 North Carothers, Franklin, TN 37064.

Davis, M., Eshelman, E. R., & McKay, M. (1988). *The relaxation and stress reduction workbook.* Oakland, Calif.: New Harbinger.

Fanning, P. (1988). *Visualization for change.* Oakland, Calif.: New Harbinger.

Hirshaut, Y., & Pressman, P. I. (1992). *Breast cancer: The complete book.* New York: Bantam Books.

Locke, S., & Colligan, D. (1987). *The healer within.* New York: Mentor.

Love, S. M., & Lindsey, K. (1990). *Dr. Susan Love's breast book.* Reading, Mass.: Addison-Wesley.

Morra, M., & Potts, E. (1987). *Choices: Realistic alternatives in cancer treatment*. New York: Avon Books.

*Mullan, F., & Hoffman, B. (Eds.). (1990). *Charting the journey: An almanac of practical resources for cancer survivors*. Mount Vernon, N.Y.: Consumers Union.

Moyers, B. (1993). *Healing and the mind*. New York: Doubleday.

Rico, G. (1991). *Pain and possibility: Writing your way through personal crisis*. Los Angeles: Tarcher.

Seligman, M.E.P. (1990). *Learned optimism*. New York: Pocket Books.

*Simonton, O. C., Matthews-Simonton, S., & Creighton, J. L. (1992). *Getting well again*. New York: Bantam Books.

Smith, J. C. (1986). *Meditation*. Champaign, Ill.: Research Press.

*Winograd, S. (1992). *Get help, get positive, get well*. Highland City, Fla.: Rainbow Books.

For Cancer Survivors

*Anderson, G. (1993). *50 essential things to do when the doctor says it's cancer*. New York: Viking Penguin.

Doka, K. J. (1993). *Living with life-threatening illness*. New York: Macmillan.

Kane, J. (1991). *Be sick well*. Oakland, Calif.: New Harbinger.

LeShan, L. (1989). *Cancer as a turning point*. New York: Viking Penguin.

Lord, J. H. (1992). *Beyond sympathy*. Ventura, Calif.: Pathfinder Publishing of California.

McWilliams, J., & McWilliams, P. (1991). *You can't afford the luxury of a negative thought*. Los Angeles: Prelude Press.

Mayer, M. (1993). *Examining myself*. Boston: Faber & Faber.

Noyes, D. D., & Melody, P. (1988). *Beauty and cancer*. Los Angeles: AC Press.

Rollin, B. (1976). *First you cry*. New York: HarperCollins.

Rosenblum, D. (1993). *A time to hear, a time to help*. New York: Free Press.

Schlossberg, N. K. (1994). *Coping with life's ups and downs*. Lexington, Mass.: Lexington Books.

Siegel, B. S. (1990). *Peace, love, and healing*. New York: Harper-Collins.

Siegel, B. S. (1993). *How to live between office visits*. New York: HarperCollins.

Spiegel, D. (1993). *Living beyond limits: New hope and help for facing life-threatening illness*. New York: Times Books.

Stearns, A. K. (1984). *Living through personal crisis*. New York: Ballantine Books.

Utian, W. H., & Jacobowitz, R. S. (1990). *Managing your menopause*. New York: Simon & Schuster.

Wadler, J. (1992). *My breast*. Reading, Mass.: Addison-Wesley.

For Children

Holden, L. D. (1989). *Gran Gran's best trick: A story for children who have lost someone they love*. New York: Brunner/Mazel.

Kohlenberg, S. (1993). *Sammy's mommy has cancer*. New York: Magination Press.

Mills, J. C. (1992). *Little tree: A story for children with serious medical problems*. New York: Brunner/Mazel.

Mills, J. C. (1993). *Gentle willow: A story for children about dying*. New York: Brunner/Mazel.

van den Berg, M. (1994). *The three birds: A story for children about the loss of a loved one*. New York: Brunner/Mazel.

Resource D: Additional Sources of Help and Information

American Cancer Society (1599 Clifton Road, Atlanta, GA 30329; 404-320-3333). This nationwide organization has many local branches that offer a wide range of support services. These include Reach to Recovery, for people who have had surgery for breast cancer; Cansurmount; the Leukemia Society; the United Cancer Council; Make Today Count; and support groups for people with specific types of cancer or specific problems related to cancer such as laryngectomies. This is the first place to start for people who have been diagnosed with cancer and are seeking support.

BMT Newsletter (1985 Spruce Avenue, Highland Park, IL 60035; 708-831-1913). This newsletter contains information and personal stories about bone marrow transplants.

Cancer Care (1180 Avenue of the Americas, New York, NY 10036; 212-221-3300). This organization provides counseling and support groups at no charge as well as transportation to medical appointments and financial assistance to people with cancer who meet their guidelines.

Cancer Connection (4410 Main Street, Kansas City, MO 64111; 816-932-8453). This organization provides hotline services that will match newly diagnosed cancer patients with those who have been cured or are in remission. It also offers printed information.

Candlelighters Childhood Cancer Foundation (7910 Woodmont Avenue, Suite 460, Bethesda, MD 20814; 301-657-8401). This well-known nationwide organization provides a broad range of services to children with cancer in all stages of the disease as well as to their families. Some chapters have youth groups for siblings.

Children's Oncology Camps of America (217-793-3949). This organization publishes an annual directory of children's oncology camps throughout the United States.

The Compassionate Friends (TCF) (P.O. Box 3696, Oak Brook, IL 60522; 708-990-0010). This nationwide organization includes many local branches and offers support groups for parents who have experienced the death of a child.

Department of Vocational Rehabilitation. Each region of the country has an office of rehabilitation associated with the government. These services can provide counseling, testing, and training as well as help in job seeking to people whose career options are limited by a physical disability. This is a particularly valuable service for people who cannot return to their previous jobs because of the impact of cancer and its treatment.

Gilda's Club (195 West Houston Street, New York, NY 10014; 212-647-9700). Named for television comedian Gilda Radner, this nonresidential clubhouse provides a place where people with cancer and their families and friends can share feelings and experiences.

Let's Face It (P.O. Box 711, Concord, MA 01742; 508-371-3186). This organization provides mutual support and information to people who have facial disfigurement.

Leukemia Society of America, Inc. (733 Third Avenue, New York, NY 10017; 212-573-8484). The Leukemia Society and its local chapters offer financial and practical assistance, consultation, and referral to people with leukemia and other hematic cancers.

Make A Wish Foundation (4601 North 16th Street, Phoenix, AZ 85016). Along with the Sunshine Foundation (2842 Normandy Drive, Philadelphia, PA 19154) and the Dream Factory (P.O. Box 188, Hopkinsville, KY 42240), this organization seeks to grant the wishes of children with terminal illnesses.

National Alliance of Breast Cancer Organizations (NABCO) (1180 Avenue of the Americas, New York, NY 10036; 212-719-0154). NABCO serves as a source of information on breast cancer and also seeks to affect public policy related to breast cancer and its treatment.

National Brain Tumor Foundation (785 Market Street, San Francisco, CA 94103; 415-284-0208). This organization provides information and support to people with brain tumors as well as to their families. It publishes a resource guide and also raises funds to support brain tumor research.

National Cancer Institute (NCI) (Building 31, Room 10A18, Bethesda, MD 20892; 800-422-6237). This organization is a leader in the research on cancer and its treatments. The NCI offers a cancer information service that is available to the public by calling 800-4-CANCER. That service provides verbal and printed information on cancer and its treatment as well as on ways to cope with the interpersonal and other difficulties raised by cancer. NCI can make referrals to cancer treatment centers and facilities that are available to provide consultation and second opinions to physicians and people with cancer. The NCI can also help people locate organizations that provide support and information to people with specific types of cancer.

National Coalition for Cancer Survivorship (NCCS) (1010 Wayne Avenue, 5th floor, Silver Spring, MD 20910; 301-650-8868). According to this group, cancer survivorship begins with diagnosis. This group celebrates survival and provides resources and information to help people maintain that survival as long and as optimistically as possible. A magazine published by the NCCS is a very useful source of information on cancer and its treatment.

National Hospice Organization (1901 North Moore Street, Suite 901, Arlington, VA 22209; 703-243-5900). This is a referral service for people with terminal illnesses, providing hospice care and guidelines to facilitate caring for people who are terminally ill.

National Lymphedema Network (2211 Post Street, Suite 404, San Francisco, CA 94115; 800-541-3259). This resource center provides information about the prevention and treatment of lymphedema as well as about local support groups for people concerned about lymphedema, a swelling that is a common complication of lymph-node surgery.

National Marrow Donor Program (3433 Broadway Street N.E., Suite 400, Minneapolis, MN 55413; 800-654-1247). This is a service designed to help people identify potential marrow donors.

Patient Advocates for Advanced Cancer Treatment (PAACT) (1143 Parmelee N.W., Grand Rapids, MI 49504; 616-453-1477). This is a national organization that provides information on diagnosis, treatment, and monitoring of prostate cancer.

Physicians Data Query (PDQ). This computerized data bank provides medical information about cancer as well as about other diseases. Many university, governmental, and professional libraries offer public access to the data bank, or a PDQ search may be requested through the Cancer Information Service offered by the National Cancer Institute.

Society for the Right to Die (250 West 57th Street, New York, NY 10107; 212-246-6973). This group is an excellent source of information and forms for people who want to make living wills or assign durable power of attorney. These steps are important not only for people with cancer but also for others who want to have some control over the way they die.

Surviving! (Stanford University Medical Center, Patient Resource Center, Room H0103, Division of Radiation Oncology, 300 Pasteur Drive, Stanford, CA 94305). This is a support group for cancer survivors that publishes a useful newsletter; its services are offered through Stanford University Hospital.

Y-Me National Organization for Breast Cancer Information and Support (18220 Harwood Avenue, Homewood, IL 60430; 800-221-2141). This nationwide group offers a newsletter with information on breast cancer and also serves as an advocacy organization to encourage needed legislation and funding in this area. Local chapters provide peer support and informative programs.

References

Adams, J. (1991). Family crisis intervention and psychosocial care for children and adolescents. In C. S. Austad & W. H. Berman (Eds.), *Psychotherapy in managed health care* (pp. 111–125). Washington, D.C.: American Psychological Association.

Agnetti, G., & Young, J. (1993). Chronicity and the experience of timelessness: An intervention model. *Family Systems Medicine, 11*(1), 67–81.

Alberti, R. E., & Emmons, M. L. (1990). *Your perfect right.* San Luis Obispo, Calif.: Impact.

American Psychiatric Association. (1994). *Diagnostic and statistical manual of mental disorders* (4th ed.). Washington, D.C.: Author.

Andersen, B. L. (1992). Psychological interventions for cancer patients to enhance the quality of life. *Journal of Consulting and Clinical Psychology, 60*(4), 552–568.

Andersen, B. L., Kiecolt-Glaser, J. K., & Glaser, R. (1994). A biobehavioral model of cancer stress and disease course. *American Psychologist, 5,* 389–404.

Andrykowski, M. A., & Jacobson, P. B. (1993). Anticipatory nausea and vomiting with cancer chemotherapy. In W. Breitbart & J. C. Holland (Eds.), *Psychiatric aspects of symptom management in cancer patients* (pp. 107–128). Washington, D.C.: American Psychiatric Press.

Anholt, U. V., Fritz, G. K., & Keener, M. (1993). Self-concept in survivors of childhood and adolescent cancer. *Journal of Psychosocial Oncology, 11*(1), 1–16.

Baron, P. H. (1985). Group work with cancer patients. *Pratt Institute Creative Arts Therapy Review, 6,* 22–36.

Barraclough, J. (1994). *Cancer and emotion.* New York: Wiley.

Bauman, L. J., Gervey, R., & Siegel, K. (1992). Factors associated with cancer patients' participation in support groups. *Journal of Psychosocial Oncology, 10*(3), 1–20.

Bearison, D. J., Sadow, A. J., Granowetter, L., & Winkel, G. (1993). Patients' and parents' causal attributions for childhood cancer. *Journal of Psychosocial Oncology, 11*(3), 47–61.

Beck, A. T., Rush, A. J., Shaw, B. F., & Emery, G. (1979). *Cognitive therapy of depression.* New York: Guilford Press.

Beckham, J. C., & Godding, P. R. (1990). Sexual dysfunction in cancer patients. *Journal of Psychosocial Oncology, 8*(1), 1–16.

Beisecker, A. E., & Moore, W. P. (1994). Oncologists' perceptions of the effects of cancer patients' companions on physician-patient interactions. *Journal of Psychosocial Oncology, 12*($\frac{1}{2}$), 23–39.

Benson, H. (1979). *The mind/body effect.* New York: Simon & Schuster.

Berkman, L. F., & Breslow, L. (1983). *Health and ways of living: The Alameda County study.* New York: Oxford University Press.

Berkman, L. F., & Syme, L. S. (1979). Social networks, host resistance, and mortality: A nine-year study of Alameda County residents. *American Journal of Epidemiology, 109,* 186–204.

Bernstein, J., & Rudman, M. (1989). *Books to help children cope with separation and loss: An annotated bibliography.* Vol. 3. New Providence, N.J.: Bowker.

Bertolone, S. J., & Scott, P. (1990). The cancer educator as role model: A means of initiating attitude change. In A. Blitzer, A. H., Kutscher, S. C. Klagsbrun, R. De Bellis, F. E. Selder, I. B. Seeland, & M. Siegel (Eds.), *Communicating with cancer patients and their families* (pp. 56–59). Philadelphia: Charles Press.

Bloom, J. R., Kang, S. H., & Romano, P. (1991). Cancer and stress: The effect of social support as a resource. In C. L. Cooper & M. Watson (Eds.), *Cancer and stress: Psychological, biological and coping studies* (pp. 95–124). New York: Wiley.

Bloom, J. R., Ross, R. D., & Burnell, G. (1978). The effect of social support on patient adjustment after breast surgery. *Patient Counselling and Health Education, 1,* 50–59.

Borysenko, J. (1988). *Minding the body, mending the mind.* New York: Bantam Books.

Bos-Branolte, G. (1987). *Psychological problems in survivors of gynecologic cancers: A psychotherapeutic approach.* Oegstgeest, Netherlands: De Kempenaer.

Bowen, M. (1991). Family reaction to death. In F. Walsh & M. McGoldrick (Eds.), *Living beyond loss* (pp. 79–92). New York: Norton.

Breitbart, B. R. (1990). Factors that contribute to control and hopefulness. In A. Blitzer, A. H., Kutscher, S. C. Klagsbrun, R. De Bellis, F. E. Selder, I. B. Seeland, & M. Siegel (Eds.), *Communicating with cancer patients and their families* (pp. 26–32). Philadelphia: Charles Press.

Breitbart, W. (1989). Psychiatric management of cancer pain. *Cancer, 63* (11 suppl.), 2336–2342.

Breitbart, W., & Holland, J. C. (Eds.). (1993). *Psychiatric aspects of symptom management in cancer patients.* Washington, D.C.: American Psychiatric Press.

Breitbart, W., Levenson, J. A., & Passik, S. D. (1993). Terminally ill cancer patients. In W. Breitbart & J. C. Holland (Eds.), *Psychiatric aspects of symptom management in cancer patients* (pp. 173–230). Washington, D.C.: American Psychiatric Press.

Breitbart, W., & Passik, S. D. (1993). Psychiatric approaches to cancer pain management. In W. Breitbart & J. C. Holland (Eds.), *Psychiatric aspects of symptom management in cancer patients* (pp. 49–86). Washington, D.C.: American Psychiatric Press.

Bridge, L. R., Benson, P., Pietroni, P. C., & Priest, R. G. (1988). Relaxation and imagery in the treatment of breast cancer. *British Medical Journal, 297,* 1169–1172.

Brigham, D. D. (1994). *Imagery for getting well.* New York: Norton.

Bukberg, J., Penman, D., & Holland, J. C. (1984). Depression in hospitalized cancer patients. *Psychosomatic Medicine, 46,* 199–212.

Burbie, G. E., & Polinsky, M. L. (1992). Intimacy and sexuality after cancer treatment: Resorting a sense of wholeness. *Journal of Psychosocial Oncology, 10*(1), 19–33.

Burish, T. G., Snyder, S. J., & Jenkins, R. A. (1991). Preparing patients for cancer chemotherapy: Effect of coping preparation and relaxation interventions. *Journal of Consulting and Clinical Psychology, 59*(4), 518–525.

Burns, D. D. (1980). *Feeling good.* New York: Signet.

Call, D. A. (1990). School-based groups: A valuable support for children of cancer patients. *Journal of Psychosocial Oncology, 8*(1), 97–118.

Callan, D. B. (1989). Hope as a clinical issue in oncology social work. *Journal of Psychosocial Oncology, 7,* 31–46.

Carey, M. P., & Burish, T. G. (1987). Providing relaxation training to cancer chemotherapy patients: A comparison of three delivery techniques. *Journal of Consulting and Clinical Psychology, 55*(5), 732–737.

Carpenter, P. J. (1991). Scientific inquiry in childhood cancer psychosocial research. *Cancer, 67*(3 suppl.), 833–838.

Carpenter, P. J., Vattimo, C. J., Messbauer, L. J., Stolnitz, C., Isle, J. B.,

Stutzman, H., & Cohen, H. J. (1992). Development of a parent advocate program as part of a pediatric hematology/oncology service. *Journal of Psychosocial Oncology*, *10*(2), 27–38.

Carter, B., & McGoldrick, M. (Eds.). (1988). *The changing family life cycle*. New York: Gardner Press.

Carter, C. A., & Carter, R. E. (1994). Some observations on individual and marital therapy with breast cancer patients and spouses. *Journal of Psychosocial Oncology*, *12*($\frac{1}{2}$), 65–81.

Carter, R. E., Carter, C. A., & Siliunas, M. (1993). Marital adaptation and interaction of couples after a mastectomy. *Journal of Psychosocial Oncology*, *11*(2), 69–82.

Chandler, C. K., Holden, J. M., & Kolander, C. A. (1992). Counseling for spiritual wellness: Theory and practice. *Journal of Counseling and Development*, *71*(2), 168–175.

Chochinov, H. M. (1993). Management of grief in the cancer setting. In W. Breitbart & J. C. Holland (Eds.), *Psychiatric aspects of symptom management in cancer patients* (pp. 231–241). Washington, D.C.: American Psychiatric Press.

Christensen, D. N. (1983). Postmastectomy couple counseling: An outcome study of a structured treatment protocol. *Journal of Sexual Marital Therapy*, *9*(4), 266–275.

Combs, D. C. (1992). A death fantasy journey. *Illness, Crises and Loss*, *2*(3), 26–30.

Cooper, C. L., & Watson, M. (Eds.). (1991). *Cancer and stress: Psychological, biological and coping studies*. New York: Wiley.

Cousins, N. (1989). *Head first: The biology of hope*. New York: Dutton.

Cullinan, A. L. (1992). The social context of breast cancer within the family. In A. Blitzer, A. H. Kutscher, S. C. Klagsbrun, R. De Bellis, F. E. Selder, I. B. Seeland, & M. Siegel (Eds.), *Communicating with cancer patients and their families* (pp. 134–149). Philadelphia: Charles Press.

Cunningham, A. J., Lockwood, G. A., & Cunningham, J. A. (1991). A relationship between perceived self-efficacy and quality of life in cancer patients. *Patient Education and Counseling*, *17*, 71–78.

Cunningham, A. J., & Tocco, E. K. (1989). A randomized trial of group psychoeducational therapy for cancer patients. *Patient Education and Counseling*, *14*, 101–114.

Curbow, B., Legro, M. W., Baker, F., Wingard, J. R., & Somerfield, M. R. (1993). Loss and recovery themes of long-term survivors of bone marrow transplants. *Journal of Psychosocial Oncology*, *10*(4), 1–20.

Dakof, G. A., & Taylor, S. E. (1990). Victims' perceptions of social support: What is helpful for whom? *Journal of Personality and Social Psychology,* 58(1), 80–89.

Davis, H., IV. (1986). Effects of biofeedback and cognitive therapy on stress in patients with breast cancer. *Psychological Reports,* 59, 967–974.

Dean, C., & Hopwood, P. (1989). Liaison psychiatry in a breast cancer unit: Comment. *British Journal of Psychiatry,* 155, 98–100.

Decker, T. W., Cline-Elsen, J., & Gallagher, M. (1992). Relaxation therapy as an adjunct in radiation oncology. *Journal of Clinical Psychology,* 48(3), 388–393.

de Haes, J.C.J.M., van Knippenberg, F.C.E., & Neijt, J. P. (1990). Measuring psychological and physical distress in cancer patients: Structure and application of the Rotterdam Symptom Checklist. *British Journal of Cancer,* 62, 1034–1038.

Derogatis, L. R. (1977). *Psychological Adjustment of Illness Scale.* Baltimore: Clinical Psychometric Research.

Derogatis, L. R., Morrow, G. R., Fetting, J., Penman, D., Piasetsky, S., Schmale, A. G., Henrichs, M., & Carnicke, C. L., Jr. (1983). The prevalence of psychiatric disorders among cancer patients. *Journal of the American Medical Association,* 249, 751–757.

Doan, B. D., & Gray, R. E. (1992). The heroic cancer patient: A critical analysis of the relationship between illusion and mental health. *Canadian Journal of Behavioural Science,* 24(2), 253–266.

Doka, K. J. (1993). *Living with life-threatening illness.* New York: Macmillan.

Dropkin, M. J. (1990). Caring for the patient with head and neck cancer. In A. Blitzer, A. H. Kutscher, S. C. Klagsbrun, R. De Bellis, F. E. Selder, I. B. Seeland, & M. Siegel (Eds.), *Communicating with cancer patients and their families* (pp. 166–175). Philadelphia: Charles Press.

Edgar, L., Rosberger, Z., & Nowlis, D. (1992). Coping with cancer during the first year after diagnosis. *Cancer,* 69(3), 817–828.

Ell, K., Nishimoto, R., Mediansky, L., Mantell, J., & Hamovitch, M. (1992). Social relations, social support and survival among patients with cancer. *Journal of Psychosomatic Research,* 36(4), 531–541.

Elsenrath, D., Hettler, B., & Leafgreen, F. (1988). *Lifestyle Assessment Questionnaire.* Stevens Point, Wis.: National Wellness Institute.

Erikson, E. H. (1963). *Childhood and society.* New York: Norton.

Ettinger, R. S., & Heiney, S. P. (1993). Cancer in adolescents and young adults. *Cancer,* 71(10 suppl.), 3276–3280.

Eysenck, H. J. (1991a). Cancer and personality. In C. L. Cooper & M. Watson

(Eds.), *Cancer and stress: Psychological, biological and coping studies* (pp. 73–94). New York: Wiley.

Eysenck, H. J. (1991b). *Smoking, personality and stress: Psychosocial factors in the prevention of cancer and coronary disease.* New York: Springer-Verlag.

Fanning, P. (1988). *Visualization for change.* Oakland, Calif.: New Harbinger.

Farash, J. L. (1979). Effect of counseling on resolution of loss and body image disturbance following a mastectomy. *Dissertation Abstracts International, 39*(4), 4027.

Farrow, J. M., Cash, D. K., & Simmons, G. (1990). Communicating with cancer patients and their families. In A. Blitzer, A. H. Kutscher, S. C. Klagsbrun, R. De Bellis, F. E. Selder, I. B. Seeland, & M. Siegel (Eds.), *Communicating with cancer patients and their families* (pp. 1–17). Philadelphia: Charles Press.

Fawzy, F. I., Cousins, N., Fawzy, N. W., Kemeny, M. E., Elashoff, R., & Morton, D. (1990). A structured psychiatric intervention for cancer patients: I. Changes over time in methods of coping and affective disturbance. *Archives of General Psychiatry, 47,* 720–725.

Fawzy, F. I., Fawzy, N. W., Hyun, C. S., Elashoff, R., Guthrie, D., Fahey, J. L., & Morton, D. L. (1993). Malignant melanoma. *Archives of General Psychiatry, 50*(9), 681–689.

Fawzy, F. I., & Morton, D. (1990). A structured psychiatric intervention for cancer patients. *Archives of General Psychiatry, 47*(8), 729–735.

Fife, B. L., Kennedy, V. N., & Robinson, L. (1994). Gender and adjustment to cancer: Clinical implications. *Journal of Psychosocial Oncology, 12*($\frac{1}{2}$), 1–21.

Fischer, J., & Corcoran, K. (1994). *Measures for clinical practice.* New York: Free Press.

Flapan, D. (1986). The trauma of the therapist's illness. *Issues in Ego Psychology, 9*(2), 32–39.

Fleishman, S. B., Lesko, L. M., & Breitbart, W. (1993). Treatment of organic mental disorders in cancer patients. In W. Breitbart & J. C. Holland (Eds.), *Psychiatric aspects of symptom management in cancer patients* (pp. 23–47). Washington, D.C.: American Psychiatric Press.

Foley, K. M. (1986). The treatment of pain in the patient with cancer. *CA: A Journal for Clinicians, 36*(4), 194–215.

Folkman, S., & Lazarus, R. S. (1980). An analysis of coping in a middle-aged community sample. *Journal of Health and Social Behavior, 21,* 219–239.

Forester, B., Kornfeld, D. S., & Fleiss, J. L. (1985). Psychotherapy during radiotherapy: Effects on emotional and physical distress. *American Journal of Psychiatry, 142,* 22–27.

Frankl, V. E. (1963). *Man's search for meaning*. New York: Washington Square Press.

Friedman, L. C., Nelson, D. V., Baer, P. E., Lane, M., Smith, F. E., & Dworkin, R. J. (1992). The relationship of dispositional optimism, daily life stress, and domestic environment to coping methods used by cancer patients. *Journal of Behavioral Medicine, 15*(2), 127–141.

Fuller, S., & Swenson, C. H. (1992). Marital quality and quality of life among cancer patients and their spouses. *Journal of Psychosocial Oncology, 10*(3), 41–56.

Ganz, P. A. (1988). Patient education as a moderator of psychological distress. *Journal of Psychosocial Oncology, 6*, 181–197.

Glanu, K., & Lerman, C. (1992). Psychosocial impact of breast cancer: A critical review. *Annals of Behavioral Medicine, 14*(3), 204–212.

Golden, W. L., Gersh, W. D., & Robbins, D. M. (1992). *Psychological treatment of cancer patients*. Needham Heights, Mass.: Allyn & Bacon.

Gon, L. M. (1993). Ethnic issues affecting the provision and use of health care services among Asian patients. *Illness, Crises and Loss, 3*(2), 17–21.

Gorfinkle, K., & Redd, W. H. (1993). Behavioral control of anxiety, distress and learned aversions in pediatric oncology. In W. Breitbart & J. C. Holland (Eds.), *Psychiatric aspects of symptom management in cancer patients* (pp. 129–146). Washington, D.C.: American Psychiatric Press.

Gotcher, J. M. (1992). Interpersonal communication and psychosocial adjustment. *Journal of Psychosocial Oncology, 10*(3), 21–39.

Graves, P. L. (1990). Psychological correlates in the development of cancer. *Psychiatric Medicine, 8*(4), 23–35.

Greening, K. (1992). The "Bear Essentials" program: Helping young children and their families cope when a parent has cancer. *Journal of Psychosocial Oncology, 10*(1), 47–61.

Greer, S., & Burgess, C. (1987). A self-esteem measure for patients with cancer. *Psychology and Health, 1*, 327–340.

Greer, S., Moorey, S., Baruch, J.D.R., Watson, M., Robinson, B. M., Mason, A., Rowden, L., Law, M., & Bliss, J. M. (1992). Adjuvant psychological therapy for patients with cancer: A prospective randomised trial. *British Medical Journal, 304*, 675–680.

Greer, S., & Watson, M. (1982). Mental adjustment to cancer: Its measurement and prognostic importance. *Cancer Surveys, 6*, 439–453.

Grossarth-Maticek, R., & Eysenck, H. J. (1989). Length of survival and lymphocyte percentage in women with mammary cancer as a function of psychotherapy. *Psychological Reports, 65*(1), 315–321.

Haber, S. (Ed.). (1993). *Breast cancer: A psychological treatment manual*. Phoenix: Division of Independent Practice.

Hatfield, T., & Hatfield, S. R. (1992). As if your life depended on it: Promoting cognitive development to promote wellness. *Journal of Counseling and Development, 71*(2), 164–167.

Heim, E. (1991). Coping and adaptation in cancer. In C. L. Cooper & M. Watson (Eds.), *Cancer and stress: Psychological, biological and coping studies* (pp. 197–231). New York: Wiley.

Hislop, G. T., Waxler, N. E., Coldman, A. J., Elmwood, J. M., & Kan, L. (1987). The prognostic significance of psychosocial factors in women with breast cancer. *Journal of Chronic Diseases, 40*(7), 729–735.

Holland, J. C. (1992). Psychooncology: Where are we, and where are we going. *Journal of Psychosocial Oncology, 10*(2), 103–112.

Holley, B. (1983). Counseling the head and neck cancer patient: Laryngectomy. *Progress in Clinical Biological Research, 121,* 215–225.

Hopwood, P., & Maguire, P. (1992). Priorities in the psychological care of cancer patients. *International Review of Psychiatry, 4,* 35–44.

Horowitz, S. A., & Breitbart, W. (1993). Relaxation and imagery for symptom control in cancer patients. In W. Breitbart & J. C. Holland (Eds.), *Psychiatric aspects of symptom management in cancer patients* (pp. 147–171). Washington, D.C.: American Psychiatric Press.

Hughes, J. E. (1987). Psychological and social consequences of cancer. *Cancer Surveys, 6*(3), 455–475.

Hursti, T., Fredrikson, M., Borjeson, S., Furst, C. J., Peterson, C., & Steineck, G. (1992). Association between personality characteristics and the prevalence and extinction of conditioned nausea after chemotherapy. *Journal of Psychosocial Oncology, 10*(2), 59–77.

Jacobson, P. B., & Holland, J. C. (1991). The stress of cancer: Psychological responses to diagnosis and treatment. In C. L. Cooper & M. Watson (Eds.), *Cancer and stress: Psychological, biological and coping studies* (pp. 147–169). New York: Wiley.

Jay, S. M., & Elliott, C. (1986). Acute and chronic pain in adults and children with cancer. *Journal of Consulting and Clinical Psychology, 54*(5), 601–607.

Jensen, A. (1990). Using group process and therapeutic metaphor in the psychosocial care of pediatric cancer patients and their siblings. In A. Blitzer, A. H. Kutscher, S. C. Klagsbrun, R. De Bellis, F. E. Selder, I. B. Seeland, & M. Siegel (Eds.), *Communicating with cancer patients and their families*. Philadelphia: Charles Press.

Jevne, R. F. (1988). Creating stillpoints: Beyond a rational approach to counseling cancer patients. *Journal of Psychosocial Oncology, 5*(3), 1–15.

Jevne, R. F. (1990). Looking back to look ahead: A retrospective study of referrals to a cancer counselling service. *International Journal for the Advancement of Counselling, 13*, 61–72.

Kane, J. (1991). *Be sick well.* Oakland, Calif.: New Harbinger.

Kaplan, J. S. (1992). A neglected issue: The sexual side effects of current treatments for breast cancer. *Journal of Sex and Marital Therapy, 18*, 3–19.

Kash, K. M., & Breitbart, W. (1993). The stress of caring for cancer patients. In W. Breitbart & J. C. Holland (Eds.), *Psychiatric aspects of symptom management in cancer patients* (pp. 243–260). Washington, D.C.: American Psychiatric Press.

Kiecolt-Glaser, J. K., Garner, W., Speicher, C., Penn, G. M., Holliday, J., & Glaser, R. (1984). Psychosocial modifiers of immunocompetence in medical students. *Psychosomatic Medicine, 46*, 7–14.

Knakal, J. (1988). A couples group in oncology social work practice: An innovative modality. *Dynamic Psychotherapy, 6*, 153–156.

Kneier, A. W., & Temoshok, L. (1984). Repressive coping reactions in patients with malignant melanoma as compared to cardiovascular disease patients. *Journal of Psychosomatic Research, 28*, 145–155.

Kobasa, S. C. (1979). Stressful life events, personality, and health. *Journal of Personality and Social Psychology, 37*(1), 1–11.

Kübler-Ross, E. (1981). *Living with death and dying.* New York: Macmillan.

Kumar, L. (1987). Psychological supportive care in cancer patients: A review. *Indian Journal of Clinical Psychology, 14*(1), 52–55.

Labrecque, M. S., Blanchard, C. G., Ruckdeschel, J. C., & Blanchard, E. B. (1991). The impact of family presence on the physician-cancer patient interaction. *Social Science and Medicine, 33*(11), 1253–1261.

Leinster, S. J., Ashcroft, J. J., Slade, P. D., & Dewey, M. E. (1989). Mastectomy versus conservative surgery: Psychosocial effects of the patient's choice of treatment. *Journal of Psychosocial Oncology, 7*($\frac{1}{2}$), 179–192.

LeShan, L. (1966). An emotional life-history pattern associated with neoplastic disease. *Annals of the New York Academy of Sciences, 125*, 780–793.

LeShan, L. (1989). *Cancer as a turning point.* New York: Viking Penguin.

Leventhal-Belfer, L., Bakker, A. M., & Russo, C. L. (1993). Parents of childhood cancer survivors: A descriptive look at their concerns and needs. *Journal of Psychosocial Oncology, 11*(2), 19–41.

Levy, S. M., Haberman, R. B., Whiteside, T., Sanzo, K., Lee, J., & Kirkwood, J. (1990). Perceived support and tumor estrogen/progesterone receptor status as predictors of natural killer cell activity in breast cancer patients. *Psychosomatic Medicine, 52*, 73–85.

Lewis, J. A., Sperry, L., & Carlson, J. (1993). *Health counseling*. Pacific Grove, Calif.: Brooks/Cole.

Linn, M. W., Linn, B. S., & Harris, R. (1982). Effects of counseling for late stage cancer patients. *Cancer, 49*(2), 1048–1055.

Locke, S. E., & Colligan, D. (1987). *The healer within*. New York: Mentor.

Lowery, B. J., Jacobson, B. S., & DuCette, J. (1993). Causal attribution, control, and adjustment to breast cancer. *Journal of Psychosocial Oncology, 10*(4), 37–53.

Lynn, R. (1986). Repetitive existential plight: The emotional impact of recurrent serious illness. *Loss, Grief, and Care, 1*($\frac{1}{2}$), 45–52.

Macaskill, A., & Monach, J. H. (1990). Coping with childhood cancer: The case for long-term counselling help for patients and their families. *British Journal of Guidance and Counselling, 18*(1), 13–27.

McDaniel, S. H., Hepworth, J., & Doherty, W. (1992). *Medical family therapy*. New York: Basic Books.

McEvoy, M. D. (1990). When your dying becomes my dying: Aspects of caregiver's grief. In A. Blitzer, A. H. Kutscher, S. C. Klagsbrun, R. De Bellis, F. E. Selder, I. B. Seeland, & M. Siegel (Eds.), *Communicating with cancer patients and their families* (pp. 206–210). Philadelphia: Charles Press.

McGoldrick, M., & Gerson, R. (1985). *Genograms in family assessment*. New York: Norton.

McGoldrick, M., & Walsh, F. (1991). A time to mourn: Death and the family life cycle. In F. Walsh & M. McGoldrick (Eds.), *Living beyond loss* (pp. 30–49). New York: Norton.

McGuire, D. B. (1987). Advances in control of cancer pain. *Nursing Clinics of North America, 22*(3), 677–690.

McNair, D. M., Lorr, M., & Droppleman, L. F. (1992). *POMS manual*. San Diego, Calif.: EdITS.

McWilliams, J., & McWilliams, P. (1991). *You can't afford the luxury of a negative thought*. Los Angeles: Prelude Press.

Manne, S. L., Girasek, D., & Ambrosino, J. (1994). An evaluation of the impact of a cosmetics class on breast cancer patients. *Journal of Psychosocial Oncology, 12*($\frac{1}{2}$), 83–99.

Manne, S. L., Redd, W. H., Jacobson, P. B., Gorfinkle, K., Schorr, O., & Rapkin, B. (1990). Behavioral intervention to reduce child and parent distress during venipuncture. *Journal of Consulting and Clinical Psychology, 58*(5), 565–572.

Massie, M. J., & Holland, J. C. (1990). Depression and the cancer patient. *Journal of Clinical Psychiatry, 51*(7 suppl.), 12–19.

Massie, M. J., & Holland, J. C. (1992). The cancer patient with pain: Psychiatric complications and their management. *Journal of Pain and Symptom Management, 7*(2), 99–108.

Mathieson, C. M., & Stam, H. J. (1991). What good is psychotherapy when I am ill? Psychosocial problems and interventions with cancer patients. In C. L. Cooper & M. Watson (Eds.), *Cancer and stress: Psychological, biological and coping studies* (pp. 171–196). New York: Wiley.

Matthews, A., & Ridgeway, V. (1984). Psychological preparation for surgery. In A. Steptoe & A. Matthews (Eds.), *Health care and human behavior* (pp. 231–259). London: Academic Press.

Meichenbaum, D. (1985). *Stress inoculation training.* Elmsford, N.Y.: Pergamon Press.

Mellette, S. J. (1989). Rehabilitation issues for cancer survivors: Psychosocial challenges. *Journal of Psychosocial Oncology, 7*(4), 93–100.

Mickley, J., Soeken, K., & Belcher, A. (1992). Spiritual well-being, religiousness, and hope among women with breast cancer. *Image, 24*(4), 267–272.

Miles, M. S., & Demi, A. S. (1986). Guilt in bereaved parents. In T. A. Rando (Ed.), *Parental loss of a child* (pp. 97–118). Champaign, Ill.: Research Press.

Miller, S., Wackman, D., Nunnally, E., & Saline, C. (1982). *Straight talk.* New York: New American Library.

Millon, T., Green, C., & Meagher, R. (1982). *Millon Behavioral Health Inventory manual.* Minneapolis: National Computer Systems.

Moorey, S., & Greer, S. (1989). *Psychological therapy for patients with cancer: A new approach.* Washington, D.C.: American Psychiatric Press.

Moos, R. H., Cronkite, R. C., Billings, A. G., & Finney, J. W. (1984). *Health and Daily Living Form manual.* Palo Alto, Calif.: Social Ecology Laboratory, Stanford University Medical Centers.

Moyers, B. (1993). *Healing and the mind.* New York: Doubleday.

Mullan, F., & Hoffman, B. (Eds.). (1990). *Charting the journey: An almanac of practical resources for cancer survivors.* Mount Vernon, N.Y.: Consumers Union.

Mullen, P. M., Smith, R. M., & Hill, E. W. (1993). Sense of coherence as a mediator of stress for cancer patients and spouses. *Journal of Psychosocial Oncology, 11*(3), 23–46.

Newberry, B. H., Gordon, T. L., & Meehan, S. M. (1991). Animal studies of stress and cancer. In C. L. Cooper & M. Watson (Eds.), *Cancer and stress: Psychological, biological and coping studies.* New York: Wiley.

Norman, A. D., & Brandeis, L. (1992). Addressing the needs of survivors: An action research approach. *Journal of Psychosocial Oncology, 10*(1), 3–18.

Oktay, J. S., & Walter, C. A. (1991). *Breast cancer in the life cycle: Women's experiences*. New York: Springer.

Palombi, B. J. (1992). Psychosomatic properties of wellness instruments. *Journal of Counseling and Development, 71*(2), 221–225.

Parker, D. F., Levinson, W., Mullooly, J. P., & Frymark, S. L. (1989). Using the Quality of Life Index in a cancer rehabilitation program. *Journal of Psychosocial Oncology, 7*(3), 47–62.

Payne, S. C. (1989). Anxiety and depression in women with advanced cancer: Implications for counselling. *Counselling Psychology Quarterly, 2,* 337–344.

Pennebaker, J. W. (1990). *Opening up: The healing power of confiding in others*. New York: Morrow.

Phelps, S., & Austin, N. (1987). *The assertive woman*. San Luis Obispo, Calif.: Impact.

Pine, V. R., & Brauer, C. (1986). Parental grief: A synthesis of theory, research, and intervention. In T. A. Rando (Ed.), *Parental loss of a child* (pp. 59–96). Champaign, Ill.: Research Press.

Rando, T. A. (1986a). Death of the adult child. In T. A. Rando (Ed.), *Parental loss of a child* (pp. 221–238). Champaign, Ill.: Research Press.

Rando, T. A. (1986b). Parental bereavement: An exception to the general conceptualizations of mourning. In T. A. Rando (Ed.), *Parental loss of a child* (pp. 45–58). Champaign, Ill.: Research Press.

Rando, T. A. (1986c). The unique issues and impact of the death of a child. In T. A. Rando (Ed.), *Parental loss of a child* (pp. 5–43). Champaign, Ill.: Research Press.

Rawnsley, M. A. (1990). Adapting time-limited therapy to the care of persons with cancer. In A. Blitzer, A. H. Kutscher, S. C. Klagsbrun, R. De Bellis, F. E. Selder, I. B. Seeland, & M. Siegel (Eds.), *Communicating with cancer patients and their families* (pp. 200–205). Philadelphia: Charles Press.

Redd, W. H. (1988). Behavioral approaches to treatment-related distress. *CA: A Cancer Journal for Clinicians, 38*(3), 138–145.

Redd, W. H., & Jacobson, P. B. (1988). Emotions and cancer. *Cancer, 62*(8 suppl.), 1871–1879.

Redd, W. H., Jacobson, P. B., Die-Trill, M., Dermatis, H., McEvoy, M., & Holland, J. C. (1987). Cognitive/attentional distraction in the control of conditioned nausea in pediatric cancer patients receiving chemotherapy. *Journal of Consulting and Clinical Psychology, 55*(3), 391–395.

Rico, G. (1991). *Pain and possibility: Writing your way through personal crisis*. Los Angeles: Tarcher.

Rolland, J. S. (1994). *Families, illness, and disability*. New York: Basic Books.

Rollin, B. (1976). *First you cry*. New York: HarperCollins.

Rose, J. H. (1993). Interactions between patients and providers: An exploratory study of age differences in emotional support. *Journal of Psychosocial Oncology, 11*(2), 43–67.

Rosen, E. J. (1990). *Families facing death*. Lexington, Mass.: Lexington Books.

Rossi, E. L. (1993). *The psychobiology of mind-body healing*. New York: Norton.

Royse, D., & Dhooper, S. (1988). Social services with cancer patients and their families: Implications for independent social workers. *Journal of Independent Social Work, 2*(3), 63–71.

Sabbioni, M. E. (1991). Cancer and stress: A possible role for psychoneuroimmunology in cancer research? In C. L. Cooper & M. Watson (Eds.), *Cancer and stress: Psychological, biological and coping studies* (pp. 3–26). New York: Wiley.

Sales, E. (1991). Psychosocial impact of the phase of cancer on the family: An updated review. *Journal of Psychosocial Oncology, 9*(4), 1–18.

Sales, E., Schultz, R., & Biegel, D. (1992). Predictors of strain in families of cancer patients: A review of the literature. *Journal of Psychosocial Oncology, 10*(2), 1–26.

Schag, C. C., Heinrich, R. L., & Ganz, P. A. (1983). Cancer inventory of problem situations: An instrument for assessing cancer patients' rehabilitation needs. *Journal of Psychosocial Oncology, 1*, 11–24.

Schlossberg, N. K. (1984). *Counseling adults in transition*. New York: Springer.

Schover, L. R., Evans, R. B., & von Eschenbach, A. C. (1987). Sexual rehabilitation in a cancer center: Diagnosis and outcome in 384 consultations. *Archives of Sexual Behavior, 16*(6), 445–461.

Schover, L. R., & Fife, M. (1986). Sexual counseling of patients undergoing radical surgery for pelvic or genital cancer. *Journal of Psychosocial Oncology, 3*, 21–41.

Selfridge, C. E. (1990). The impact of group counseling on the terminally ill. In A. Blitzer, A. H. Kutscher, S. C. Klagsbrun, R. De Bellis, F. E. Selder, I. B. Seeland, & M. Siegel (Eds.), *Communicating with cancer patients and their families* (pp. 192–199). Philadelphia: Charles Press.

Seligman, L. (1990a). *Selecting effective treatments: A comprehensive, systematic guide to treating adult mental disorders*. San Francisco: Jossey-Bass.

Seligman, M.E.P. (1990b). *Learned optimism*. New York: Pocket Books.

Selye, H. (1976). *The stress of life*. New York: McGraw-Hill.

Shapiro, P. A., & Kornfeld, D. S. (1987). Psychiatric aspects of head and neck cancer surgery. *Psychiatric Clinics of North America, 10*(1), 87–100.

Shekelle, R. B., Raynor, W. J., & Ostfeld, A. M. (1981). Psychological depression and 17-year risk of death from cancer. *Psychosomatic Medicine*, *43*, 117–125.

Siebert, A. (1993). *The survivor personality*. Portland, Oreg.: Practical Psychology Press.

Siegel, B. S. (1990). *Peace, love, and healing*. New York: HarperCollins.

Siegel, B. S. (1993). *How to live between office visits*. New York: HarperCollins.

Simonton, O. C., Matthews-Simonton, S., & Creighton, J. L. (1992). *Getting well again*. New York: Bantam Books.

Sitarz, A. (1990). Clinical cancer education in the pediatric setting. In A. Blitzer, A. H. Kutscher, S. C. Klagsbrun, R. De Bellis, F. E. Selder, I. B. Seeland, & M. Siegel (Eds.), *Communicating with cancer patients and their families* (pp. 49–55). Philadelphia: Charles Press.

Smith, D. C., Richards, W., & Maher, M. F. (1993). Metaphoric language: Palliation for the terminally ill. *Illness, Crises and Loss*, *2*(4), 38–44.

Smith, J. C. (1986). *Meditation*. Champaign, Ill.: Research Press.

Sourkes, B. M. (1991). Truth to life: Art therapy with pediatric oncology patients and their siblings. *Journal of Psychosocial Oncology*, *9*(2), 81–96.

Speechley, K. N., & Noh, S. (1992). Surviving childhood cancer, social support, and parents' psychological adjustment. *Journal of Pediatric Psychology*, *17*(1), 15–31.

Spencer, S. A., & Adams, J. D. (1990). *Life changes: Growing through personal transitions*. San Luis Obispo, Calif.: Impact.

Spiegel, D. (1985). The use of hypnosis in controlling cancer pain. *CA: A Cancer Journal for Clinicians*, *35*(4), 221–231.

Spiegel, D. (1992). Effects of psychosocial support on patients with metastatic breast cancer. *Journal of Psychosocial Oncology*, *10*(2), 113–120.

Spiegel, D., & Bloom, J. R. (1983). Group therapy and hypnosis reduce metastatic breast carcinoma pain. *Psychosomatic Medicine*, *45*, 333–339.

Spiegel, D., Bloom, J. R., & Yalom, I. D. (1981). Group support for metastatic cancer patients: A randomized prospective outcome study. *Archives of General Psychiatry*, *38*, 527–533.

Spiegel, H., & Spiegel, D. (1978). *Trance and treatment*. Washington, D.C.: American Psychiatric Press.

Stam, H. J., Koopmans, J. P., & Mathieson, C. M. (1991). The psychosocial impact of a laryngectomy: A comprehensive assessment. *Journal of Psychosocial Oncology*, *9*(3), 37–58.

Sullivan, I. (1990). Cancer: A situational problem. In A. Blitzer, A. H. Kutscher, S. C. Klagsbrun, R. De Bellis, F. E. Selder, I. B. Seeland, & M. Siegel (Eds.), *Communicating with cancer patients and their families* (pp. 60–76). Philadelphia: Charles Press.

Sutherland, H. J., Lockwood, G. A., & Cunningham, A. J. (1989). A simple, rapid method for assessing psychological distress in cancer patients: Evidence of validity for linear analog scales. *Journal of Psychosocial Oncology*, 7($\frac{1}{2}$), 31–43.

Taylor-Brown, J., Acheson, A., & Farber, J. M. (1993). Kids can cope: A group intervention for children whose parents have cancer. *Journal of Psychosocial Oncology*, 11(1), 41–53.

Telch, C. F., & Telch, M. J. (1986). Group coping skills instruction and supportive therapy for cancer patients: A comparison of strategies. *Journal of Consulting and Clinical Psychology*, 54(8), 802–808.

Temoshok, L., & Dreher, H. (1992). *The Type C connection*. New York: Random House.

Thomas, C. B., Dusynski, K. R., & Shaffer, J. W. (1979). Family attitudes in youth as potential predictors of cancer. *Psychosomatic Medicine, 41*, 287–301.

Trijsburg, R. W., van Knippenberg, F.C.E., & Rijpma, S. E. (1992). Effects of psychological treatment on cancer patients: A critical review. *Psychosomatic Medicine, 54*, 489–517.

Vachon, M.L.S. (1987). Unresolved grief in persons with cancer referred for psychotherapy. *Psychiatric Clinics of North America, 10*(3), 467–486.

van Rood, Y., & Balner, H. (Eds.). (1990). *Conceptual and methodological issues in cancer psychotherapy intervention studies*. Amsterdam: Swets & Zeitlinger.

Visintainer, M. A., Volpicelli, J. R., & Seligman, M.E.B. (1982). Tumor rejection in rats after inescapable or escapable shock. *Sciences, 216*, 437–439.

Vugia, H. D. (1991). Support groups in oncology: Building hope through the human bond. *Journal of Psychosocial Oncology, 9*(3), 89–107.

Wadler, J. (1992). *My breast*. Reading, Mass.: Addison-Wesley.

Wallston, B. S., Wallston, K. A., Kaplan, G. D., & Maides, S. A. (1976). Development and validation of the Health Locus of Control (HLC) scale. *Journal of Consulting and Clinical Psychology, 44*, 580–585.

Wallston, K. A., Wallston, B. S., & Devellis, R. (1978). Development of the Multidimensional Health Locus of Control (MHLOC) scales. *Health Education Monographs, 6*, 160–170.

Ward, S., Leventhal, H., Easterling, D., Luchterhand, C., & Love, R. (1991). Social support, self-esteem, and communication in patients receiving chemotherapy. *Journal of Psychosocial Oncology, 9*(1), 95–116.

Watson, M., Denton, S., Baum, M., & Greer, S. (1988). Counselling breast cancer patients: A specialist nurse service. *Counselling Psychology Quarterly, 1*, 25–34.

Watson, M., & Greer, S. (1983). Development of a questionnaire measure of emotional control. *Journal of Psychosomatic Research, 27*, 299–305.

Watson, M., Greer, S., Young, J., Inayat, Q., Burgess, C., & Robertson, B. (1988). Development of a questionnaire measure of adjustment to cancer: The MAC scale. *Psychological Medicine, 18,* 203–209.

Watson, M., & Ramirez, A. (1991). Psychological factors in cancer prognosis. In C. L. Cooper & M. Watson (Eds.), *Cancer and stress: Psychological, biological and coping studies* (pp. 47–71). New York: Wiley.

Westlake, S. B., & Selder, F. E. (1990). Breast cancer: Living with uncertainty. In A. Blitzer, A. H. Kutscher, S. C. Klagsbrun, R. De Bellis, F. E. Selder, I. B. Seeland, & M. Siegel (Eds.), *Communicating with cancer patients and their families* (pp. 125–133). Philadelphia: Charles Press.

Winefield, H. R., & Neuling, S. J. (1987). Social support, counselling, and cancer. *British Journal of Guidance and Counselling, 15*(1), 6–16.

Winograd, S. (1992). *Get help, get positive, get well.* Highland City, Fla.: Rainbow Books.

Witmer, J. M., Rich, C., Barcikowski, R., & Mague, J. C. (1983). Psychosocial characteristics mediating the stress response: An exploratory study. *Personnel and Guidance Journal, 62,* 73–77.

Witmer, J. M., & Sweeney, T. J. (1992). A holistic model of wellness and prevention over the life span. *Journal of Counseling and Development, 71*(2), 140–148.

Worden, J. W. (1991). *Grief counseling and grief therapy.* New York: Springer.

Zeltzer, L. K., Dolgin, M. J., Le Baron, S., & Le Baron, C. (1991). A randomized, controlled study of behavioral intervention for chemotherapy distress in children with cancer. *Pediatrics, 88*(1), 34–42.

Zigmond, A. S., & Snaith, R. P. (1983). The Hospital Anxiety and Depression (HAD) scale. *Acta Psychiatrica Scandinavica, 67,* 361–370.

Zimpfer, D. G. (1989). Groups for persons who have cancer. *Journal for Specialists in Group Work, 89,* 98–104.

Zimpfer, D. G. (1992). Psychosocial treatment of life-threatening disease: A wellness model. *Journal of Counseling and Development, 71*(2), 203–209.

Name Index

Subject Index

• •